MENOPAUSE
and the years ahead

By
Mary K. Beard, M.D., F.A.C.O.G.
and
Lindsay R. Curtis, M.D., F.A.C.O.G.

Illustrations by
Paul Farber

REVISED

FISHER BOOKS

Publishers: Fred W. Fisher
    Helen V. Fisher
    Howard W. Fisher
Editors: Joyce Bush
    Veronica Durie
    Bill Fisher
    J. McCrary
Cover Design: Josh Young
Cover Photography
 Front: Joshua JamesYoung
 Author: Busath Photography

Published by Fisher Books
P.O. Box 38040
Tucson, Arizona 85740-8040
(602) 292-9080

Library of Congress Cataloging-in-Publication Data

Beard, Mary K.
 Menopause and the years ahead / by Mary K. Beard and Lindsay R. Curtis; illustrations by Paul Farber.—Rev. ed.
 p. cm.
 Includes bibliographical references and index.
 ISBN 1-55561-043-9: $12.95
 1. Menopause. 2. Middle-age women—Health and hygiene.
I. Curtis, Lindsay R.
II. Title. years ahead.
RG186.B42 1991
612'.665—dc20   91-17421
           CIP

©1991 Fisher Books

Printed in U. S. A.
Printing 10 9 8 7

Notice: *The information in this book is true and complete to the best of our knowledge. This book is intended only as an informative guide for those wishing to know more about menopause. This book is not intended to replace, countermand or conflict with the advice given to you by your physician. He or she knows your history, symptoms, signs, allergies, general health and the many other variables that challenge his/her judgment in caring for you as a patient. The information in this book is general and is offered with no guarantees on the part of the authors or Fisher Books. The authors and publisher disclaim all liability in conjunction with the use of this book.*

Contents

About the Authors

Mary Beard, M.D., F.A.C.O.G., is a graduate of the University of Arkansas School of Medicine. She completed her residency in Obstetrics and Gynecology at Washington University, Barnes Hospital. Dr. Beard is a fellow of the American College of Obstetrics and Gynecology, a Diplomate of the American Board of Obstetrics and Gynecology and an Assistant Clinical Professor in Obstetrics and Gynecology at the University of Utah College of Medicine. She is involved in women's health-care issues and has served on many hospital committees. She has been the Medical Director of McKay-Dee's Women's Center and consultant to their PMS Center. Dr. Beard has a successful private OB-GYN and infertility practice in Salt Lake City, Utah. Prior to working in this field, she practiced internal medicine for 16 years in Hawaii. Dr. Beard co-authored the book *My Body, My Decision*. She travels extensively to lecture on menopause, osteoporosis and estrogen-replacement therapy.

Lindsay Curtis, M.D., F.A.C.O.G., has written many books dealing with women's health problems. Dr. Curtis graduated from the University of Colorado School of Medicine and is a fellow of the American College of Obstetrics and Gynecology, a Diplomate of the American Board of Obstetrics and Gynecology and an Assistant Clinical Professor at the University of Utah College of Medicine. Dr. Curtis has also served as educational consultant for the Utah Division of the American Cancer Society.

As a prominent medical writer, Dr. Curtis has written the syndicated column *For Women Only*, and is the author of the best-selling books *Pregnant and lovin' it, Sensible Sex, About My Daughter, Doctor,* and *Solving Sex Problems in Marriage.* In addition to writing numerous booklets and pamphlets used by pharmaceutical companies, the armed forces and the American Cancer Society, Dr. Curtis co-authored the books *My Body, My Decision* and *Pregnancy & Sports Fitness.*

Introduction

Menopause is inevitable—if you live long enough. And like puberty, menopause is a major change in your life and identity as you pass from a reproductive to a non-reproductive status.

You may be fortunate enough to have no unpleasant menopausal symptoms, but if you are among the 85 percent[1] who do, much can be done to relieve these symptoms safely and successfully.

Female hormones were used to treat menopausal symptoms in the 1940s and 1950s. They provided welcome relief from nervousness, insomnia, hot flashes, genito-urinary atrophy and many other menopausal symptoms that had always been taken for granted in women nearing 50.

Unfortunately the threat of breast and uterine cancer in the 1960s and 1970s cast a shadow over the use of hormones. Once again those women with severe menopausal symptoms were left to suffer with little hope of relief. Extensive research has exonerated female sex hormones as a cause of breast cancer. It has also vindicated estrogen (when combined with progestogen) as a cause of cancer of the uterus.

Estrogen-replacement therapy (ERT) is not only safe, it is truly *lifesaving.* Whereas the relief of uncomfortable vasomotor menopausal symptoms such as hot flashes and insomnia were the prime reasons for taking ERT, research has demonstrated that ERT *must* be taken by nearly every postmenopausal woman to avoid crippling, deforming and life-threatening osteoporosis and also to prevent cardiovascular tragedies.

You can obtain safe relief from your discomfort during postmenopausal years, but it is essential to your life and health to understand *why* ERT is lifesaving to you. That's why we wrote this book—to answer all of your questions about menopause.

1   Notelovitz, M. "Estrogen Replacement Therapy: Indications, Contraindications and Agent Selection." *American Journal of Obstetrics & Gynecology.* 1989. 161:1832-41.

Dedication

Dedicated to women in and beyond the menopause to inform them that unpleasant menopausal symptoms can be relieved; that osteoporosis is a preventable disease along with its fractures and disfigurement; and that estrotogen-replacement therapy (ERT) may also help to prevent cardiovascular disease and thus prolong their lives.

1

Menopause – What It Is and Isn't

The word *menopause* means *to stop menstrual periods*. We think of menopause as not only stopping menstrual periods, but also as the end of fertility and childbearing. Menopause is often accompanied by unpleasant symptoms and physical changes.

The *climacteric* is the more correct term to describe this phase of a woman's life when she passes from the reproductive (child-bearing) years to the non-reproductive years.

Women are the only mammals that stop menstruating long before they die and lose their fertility when only two-thirds of their life is over. This is a 20th-century phenomenon because life expectancy before 1900 was only 45 to 48 years. Now women live to an average of 78 to 80 years—outliving their ovarian function by 30 years.

The average girl spends 12 to 14 years just growing up. She then becomes fertile and remains fertile for about 37 years. She may have another 30 years ahead of her during which time she will not be fertile. So why does she run out of fertility?

There are about 5-million oocytes (potential eggs) in each ovary of a 20-week-old fetus. This number is gradually reduced to 1 to 2 million at birth.

By puberty, these eggs have been reduced to 300,000 to 400,000 *ova* (eggs) in an immature form. The cells surrounding each ovum form what is called a *follicle* and produce hormones known as *estrogen* and *progesterone*. These follicles (with their eggs) are further reduced to less than 10,000 by age 45, although only 300 to 400 have actually been released during the years of monthly ovulation. Normally, only one egg is released at each ovulation.

Perhaps you are wondering what happens to the other ova that lost the race for ovulation?

These follicles gradually atrophy and lose their ability to produce estrogen. Usually by about age 50, all 400,000 eggs in each ovary have either been released with ovulation (only one per cycle) or they have atrophied (dried up). At the beginning of each menstrual cycle, 10 to 500 eggs begin to develop in each ovary. About a week into the cycle, most of the eggs are atrophying or have stopped developing. Although only one egg is released with ovulation, 20 to 1,000 eggs may be eliminated each month. When all of the ova have been used up (atrophied), estrogen production ceases and menopause occurs.

Menopause occurs when your ovaries run out of eggs and hence you run out of estrogen fluid. Or at least your level of estrogen is reduced to a point where you develop menopausal symptoms. It's true a small amount of estrogen is also produced by your adrenal glands and possibly some other tissues of your body. But the primary source of estrogen is your ovaries.

As your menstrual flow ends each month, the hypothalamus (area of brain just above pituitary gland) sends a message to the pituitary gland which then pours out a hormone that stimulates many of your follicles to grow. As the cells surrounding the ovum in these follicles grow, they produce increasing amounts of estrogen which in turn stimulate the lining of the uterus to grow (thicken).

At the same time the cells of the follicle are growing, the ovum inside the follicle is maturing and the follicle is moving toward the surface of the ovary. The first ovum to mature and reach the surface of the ovary is released, a process called *ovulation*. This is the egg that will find itself drawn into the fallopian tube and propelled toward the uterine cavity. While within the fallopian tube, this egg may encounter a sperm, become fertilized, then continue to the uterine cavity, become implanted and develop into a fetus (baby).

After releasing its ovum, the remaining follicle and its cells grow as they produce (under the influence of another hormone from the hypothalamus-pituitary complex) progesterone, a hormone which further prepares the lining of the uterus for implantation of the fertilized ovum. This follicle, now greatly increased in size, is known as the *corpus luteum of pregnancy*. It produces sufficient progesterone to maintain the pregnancy until the placenta and its hormone take over this task at a later date.

ક્ષ   ક્ષ   ક્ષ

It is not unusual to have symptoms of bladder dysfunction when there is estrogen deficiency.

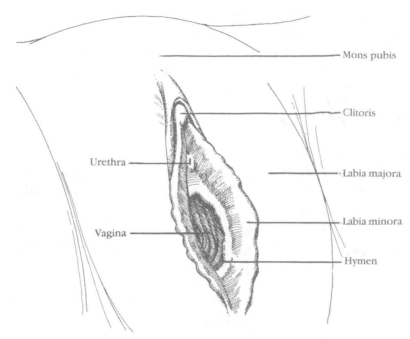

Mons pubis

Clitoris

Urethra

Labia majora

Labia minora

Vagina

Hymen

Vulva and external female organs.

If pregnancy does not occur, this follicle will become the *corpus luteum of menstruation*. It begins to regress about 1 week before the menses and slowly atrophies (dries up).[1]

- *What is ERT?*

  ERT are the letters that indicate Estrogen Replacement Therapy. When progesterone is also included, some refer to this as HRT or Hormone Replacement Therapy, but generally ERT is used to cover either method. Synthetically produced progesterones are called *progestogens* or *progestins*.

- *What is the difference between menopause and climacteric?*

  Theoretically, *menopause* means simply the stopping of menstrual periods. *Climacteric* refers to the entire phase of declining ovarian function. This phase may include several years prior to menopause plus a few years afterward.

- *At what age does menopause usually occur?*

  Menopause occurs between 48 and 52, but may start as early as

---

1 Baker, T.C. "Development of the Ovary and Oogenesis." *Clinical Obstetrics & Gynecology.* 1976. 3:26.

the late 30s and as late as the mid-50s. The average age seems to be increasing only slightly. It does not seem to be related to better nutrition, the use of oral contraceptives, the age of onset of menses or even the number of children born.

The age at which your menopause occurs is genetically predetermined. It will probably be close to the age at which your mother had her menopause.

- *How long does menopause last?*

Menstrual periods stop abruptly in some women. In others, the menstrual periods gradually decrease over a period of months or even longer.

A waxing and waning of menstrual flow over a year or two causes some women to worry about cancer of the lining of the uterus. A biopsy of the endometrium (lining of the uterus) or a D&C (scraping of the inner lining of the uterus) may be necessary to rule out cancer when irregular bleeding occurs. Pages 32–36.

Other symptoms of the climacteric may begin months before the menses stop and persist for a short time—or extend off and on for the rest of a woman's life. Example: vaginal and bladder atrophy (thinning and shrinking) develop slowly and get worse with age. Some women report occasional hot flashes into their 80s.

- *Does every woman have unpleasant symptoms during menopause?*

No. About 15 percent of women have few or no symptoms; about the same number experience severe symptoms. The most common symptom is the hot flash and 75% to 85% of women experience them during the climacteric.[2]

- *Are those menopausal symptoms just in my head?*

Definitely not! While it is true some of the symptoms are related to your emotional state, they are *not* imaginary.

Menopause symptoms are divided into three categories:

2 Bates, G.W. "On the Nature of the Hot Flash." *Clinical Obstetrics and Gynecology.* 1981. 24:231-241.

1. Autonomic (involuntary symptoms)

hot flushes

hot flashes

cold chills

angina pectoris (chest pain)

palpitations of the heart

night sweats

increased perspiration

2. Physical and metabolic changes

menstrual changes

changes in cycle (shorten or lengthen)

changes in flow amount (increase or decrease)

breast-size decrease (atrophy)

skin thinning and wrinkling (atrophy)

vaginal atrophy (dryness, burning, itching)

discharge and occasional bleeding

dyspareunia (painful intercourse)

contracting and scarring of tissues

shortening and narrowing

vaginal relaxation with prolapsing (falling out of position)

increased facial, chest and abdominal hair

bladder dysfunction

frequency of urination

dysuria (burning or stinging sensation when passing urine)

increased bladder infection

bladder infection symptoms without infection

osteoporosis

increased muscular weakness

degeneration of bone joints

increased cardiovascular disease (heart attacks and strokes)

3. Psychogenic

apathy

apprehension

decline in libido

depression

fatigue

forgetfulness

formication (feeling like ants under the skin)

frigidity

headaches

insomnia

irritability

mood changes

We can almost immediately relieve most or all of the autonomic or involuntary symptoms with estrogen. There's simply no reason why you should suffer from any of these symptoms. It may take a little fine tuning to determine the exact amount of estrogen you require, but you can be assured of relief.

Studies have shown an increase in finger temperatures and skin temperatures corresponding with fluctuations in plasma hormone levels when you have a hot flash. In other words, they are real and have a physiological basis.

Physical and metabolic changes may be slowed by ERT (estrogen-replacement therapy). But these symptoms will continue to a certain extent. Because many of these changes are due to aging, they cannot be totally blamed upon menopause.

Thinning and wrinkling of your skin, for instance, will continue but possibly at a slower rate on ERT. Some evidence suggests estrogen has a beneficial effect upon collagen, the connective tissue under the skin. Some researchers believe estrogen slows the loss of collagen from the skin and may slow the wrinkling process in your skin.[3]

Vaginal atrophy and bladder symptoms are relieved by estrogen. The tissue in the urethra and bladder area are *estrogen-dependent.*

Normally estrogen increases breast size, but only temporarily and is not prescribed for this purpose.

Degeneration of joints may progress, but at a slower pace when taking estrogen.

Unless other causes are present, the psychogenic symptoms due to menopause are relieved by ERT. Recent studies indicate irritability accompanying menopause may be connected with loss of sleep. If you lose some sleep each night, it is similar to a daily overdraft in your bank balance. Eventually it catches up with you.

Fatigue and irritability are related to sleep deprivation, so ERT may relieve both of these symptoms. Loss of sleep is often due to hot flashes that interrupt or prevent REM (normal, restful) sleep patterns, without which you will awaken tired and unrested.[4]

ðŸ™‚   ðŸ™‚   ðŸ™‚

ERT is Estrogen Replacement Therapy. When progestogen is included, some refer to this as HRT or Hormone Replacement Therapy.

3   Brincat, M. et al. "A Study of the Decrease of Skin Collagen, Skin Thickness and Bone Mass in the Postmenopausal Woman." *Abstract of Gynecology.* 1987:70:40-45.
4   Ravnikar, V.A. et al. "Hormone Therapy for Menopausal Sleep Problems." *Contemporary OB/Gyn.* 1990. 75:53S.

Also estrogen has a definite effect on certain chemicals in the brain that are associated with depression. Decrease or total loss of estrogen during menopause could be a reason for depressive feelings.[5]

These symptoms are not in your head. They are not imaginary. And they can be relieved!

- *What should I expect during menopause?*

  Be well informed. Climacteric symptoms vary widely in different women. Don't compare your symptoms with someone else's. Expect some symptoms (85 percent of women do), but know you can obtain excellent relief from all symptoms.

  Because of estrogen-replacement therapy (ERT), it is no longer necessary for most women to suffer during menopause.

- *Can you tell me more about hot flashes and what causes them?*

  A hot flash is a sudden feeling of heat throughout your upper body. It may be apparent to others only in your face and neck. Your face may flush and develop beads of perspiration—even in a cold room. This warm feeling is due to the dilation (filling) of the capillaries next to your skin.

  If this happens at night, as flashes often do, you may awaken to find your bed sheets soaking wet from perspiration. Fat women have a more severe experience than thin women, perhaps because of their greater body surface.

  Your skin temperature actually elevates during a flash. Perhaps this is why your flash may be followed by a chilling sensation. You may or may not feel a hot flash coming on before it occurs.

  The hot flash is activated in the hypothalamus (part of the brain) and disturbs the thermo-regulators of your body. This chaos in your heat-regulating mechanism results in the flash and may also cause the chilling sensation that often follows.

  In certain women, exercise, hot weather, excitement or even hot drinks may provoke hot flashes, but the falling estrogen level is the culprit behind the entire process. This is why estrogen relieves hot flashes.

---

5 Shangold, M.M. "Exercise in the Menopausal Woman." *Obstetrics and Gynecology.* 1990. 75: 53S.

- *Why do some women have more severe menopausal symptoms than others?*

  We think this has to do with the rate at which estrogen is lost. This is why women who have their ovaries removed when they have a hysterectomy (before their natural menopause) have more severe menopausal symptoms unless given ERT (estrogen-replacement therapy).

  Some women receive a fair amount of estrogen from their adrenal glands, which are located on the kidneys, and also from some other organs of the body. These women may have mild or no symptoms of menopause when their ovaries cease functioning.

  The appearance and severity of menopausal symptoms have nothing to do with whether you are emotional or even hypochondriacal. These real symptoms seem to depend upon the amount of estrogen your body is producing and whether this amount of estrogen is decreasing. Even usually stoic women will complain of menopausal symptoms if they are having them.

- *What can I do about insomnia?*

  First, be sure you are taking ERT and you are checking the dosage with your doctor. Some women require more estrogen than others. If a woman is allergic to estrogen then we consider other forms of therapy. Like estrogen, progestogen prevents (and relieves) some menopausal symptoms that occur when estrogen is diminished. Skin-patch estrogen can be substituted if the problem is that your stomach can't tolerate estrogen.

  The hypothalamus is the first organ affected by a deficiency of estrogen and it is also the part of the brain that controls sleep. Hence, it is important for you to take sufficient estrogen if you are to sleep normally.

  Because estrogen levels rise to as much as 1,000 times the normal level during pregnancy then drop rapidly after delivery, it is small wonder women often have insomnia and depression due to low estrogen levels after having a baby (known as *"After-Baby Blues"*). The same mechanism may be in effect when estrogen levels drop during menopause.

  It is also important to realize depression can occur at the same time as menopause, but is not necessarily due to it. If your depression continues in spite of estrogen therapy, consult your doctor and tell him of your feelings before the depression leads to insomnia and the resultant depression becomes too severe.

- *Is weight gain a normal part of menopause?*

  It is true many women have a tendency to gain weight after menopause, regardless of ERT. As one ages the total lean-body mass (muscle) decreases and the percent of total body fat increases with a tendency to localize on the abdomen and thighs.

  It is possible your metabolism slows down and you do not burn up as many calories as you used to. Another consideration is both men and women tend to be less active as they reach midlife while continuing to eat as much. The inevitable result is weight gain.

  It is a good idea to start a practical exercise routine, whether with a spa, club, or at home. Also remember you do not require as much food as you used to. Some of this weight gain may be due to water retention. See page 160 for more discussion.

- *I am only 32 and I am having occasional hot flashes. I notice less vaginal secretion and a tendency toward dryness of my vagina during intercourse. Could I be going through early menopause?*

  Yes, but these same symptoms may also be due to stress. Women sometimes skip menstrual periods and develop menopausal symptoms when there's a death in the family, if they change climate or experience other stressful changes such as divorce or relocation. Causes of early or premature (before 35) menopause are:

  1. Autoimmune response (an allergic response to your own body chemistry). Certain poorly understood diseases such as primary hypothyroidism, thyroiditis, adrenal insufficiency, diabetes mellitus, myasthenia gravis, pernicious anemia and oophoritis are thought to be due to an autoimmune response. These conditions may provoke an early onset of menopause. Other unknown causes of decreased estrogen production can also cause premature menopause.

  2. Induced menopause. Surgical removal of the ovaries, irradiation of the ovaries and chemotherapy can also cause early menopause at whatever age these measures are taken.

  3. Heredity. If your mother or grandmother had an early menopause, it is likely you may follow their pattern.

  4. Abnormal chromosomes. These limit the number of follicles in your ovaries. As mentioned, menopause occurs when the supply of follicles (and ova) in your ovaries is exhausted. A rare condition occasionally exists in which there is an abnormally high level of gonadotropins (hormones) in your pituitary gland because your ovary is unable to release ova and estrogens. It is even possible these two conditions are interrelated.

In general, we speak in terms of premature menopause when the menstrual flow stops before 35, except when due to pregnancy.

When hormone production (estrogen) decreases earlier than normal (before 50), a loss of calcium may also occur, causing a greater risk and an earlier onset of osteoporosis. See page 224.

Lastly, you may simply have a premature but gradual decrease in estrogen production. This can occur as early as your late 30s or early 40s and slowly progresses into menopause.

Finally, yes it is possible, although uncommon, you could be starting through menopause at 32.

- *I am 42. I have had no menstrual periods for over a year and have had the usual unpleasant symptoms of menopause. Why am I experiencing these changes at my age?*

Approximately 8 percent of women go through a spontaneous early menopause. It can be hereditary. Did your mother or grandmother also have an early menopause?. You may have inherited fewer eggs or disposed of them faster than normal. Each month one egg is released or extruded from the ovaries with ovulation. Many more (from about 1 to 2 million at birth down to none after menopause) simply atrophy (dry up) after they have tried to mature first, but lose the race to the successful egg released at ovulation.

Women who have had surgery, such as a hysterectomy or even a tubal ligation that interfered with the blood supply to the ovaries, may go through an earlier menopause. Cigarette smokers experience menopause 2 years earlier than they otherwise might have.[6]

Another factor could be autoimmune disease which can cause your body to destroy your ovarian tissue. Radiation treatments and chemotherapy can also cause early menopause.

---

6 Gold, E.B. "Smoking and the Menopause." *Menopause Management.* Nov. 1990. Vol. 3, No. 3:9-11.

- *What causes menopause to come very late, such as at 58 or so?*

Heredity may be the cause of late menopause which occurs in about 1 in 20 women.

Many women are happy to see menopause come along with the relief from menstruation and pregnancy it brings. But there are reasons why a late menopause is desirable. For instance, you may retain your youthful appearance longer along with the later appearance of wrinkles. Your bladder and vagina will not be subjected to the usual drying and thinning (atrophy) of tissues with consequent painful intercourse. Your bladder muscles will be less likely to lose their tone and control, leading to loss of urine during strain, stress, laughing, sneezing and coughing.

Even more important, you will be less likely to develop osteoporosis which can cause fractures and humping of your back. You will also be less prone to heart attacks and stroke because you have these additional years of estrogen production.

About the only disadvantage of late menopause, besides the continued menstrual periods and prolonged fertility, is a slight increase in the chance of ovarian cancer. A yearly physical and pelvic examination will help in detection of this cancer. Cancer of the ovary is particularly dangerous because it reaches an advanced state before any symptoms become evident.

- *I am 41 years old. I am having hot flashes even though I am still menstruating. Is this normal?*

This may indicate a decrease in your estrogen—but not enough to stop your menstrual periods. If your FSH (follicle-stimulating hormone) blood level proves to be high, you may need to take supplementary estrogen under your doctor's direction.

- *How soon may I expect relief from menopausal symptoms if I take estrogen-replacement therapy?*

In general, relief from flashes, nervousness and insomnia may be immediate with ERT. Improvement in your vaginal mucous membranes may be slower to appear, requiring as much as several weeks or even up to two years.

- *I do not like to take medicine of any kind. How serious is it if I choose not to take ERT now I am past menopause?*

First of all, you are not alone. Only about 50 percent of women for whom ERT is prescribed continue to take the medicine. In fact, it is estimated only 10 to 15 percent of postmenopausal women in the United States take ERT.[7]

Two reasons for giving careful consideration to taking ERT are:
1. To treat the symptoms of hot flashes and genitourinary atrophy (progressive drying and thinning of the vagina and bladder).
2. To prevent osteoporosis and cardiovascular disease.

You must be the judge as to whether you want to take a chance of developing these diseases and having to live with the symptoms of the ongoing changes from a lack of estrogen.[8]

• *Are vitamins effective in relieving menopausal symptoms?*

There are those who contend vitamin B complex and vitamins C and E relieve symptoms. It is sometimes difficult to assess this relief. These vitamins taken in moderation won't hurt you, but we cannot guarantee they will relieve your symptoms.

• *What should a woman do for hot flashes if she cannot take estrogen for some reason?*

If a woman cannot take estrogen by mouth, perhaps she can use the skin-patch method.

Progestogens alone have been found to give relief to some women, especially relief from hot flashes.[9] However, the relief is about 80% as effective as estrogen and it will not protect against vaginal atrophy or cardiovascular disease.

If you decide to use tranquilizers, remember they are habit-forming and must be carefully controlled. They can only be used for a limited time and will not protect against degeneration resulting from estrogen deficiency.

Clonidine (Catapres®) is normally used to control hypertension but has also been found to relieve hot flashes.[10] It may be helpful for women who cannot take estrogen, but it will not protect

7 Ravnikar, V.A. "Compliance with Hormone Therapy" *American Journal of Obstetrics and Gynecology.* 1987. 156:1332-4.
8 Utian, W.H. "Biosynthesis and Physiologic Effects of Estrogen and the Pathophysiologic Effects of Estrogen Deficiency: A Review." *American Journal of Obstetrics and Gynecology.* 1989. 161:1828-31.
9 Schiff, I. et al. "Oral Medroxyprogesterone in the Treatment of Postmenopausal Symptoms." *Journal of the American Medical Association.* 1980. 244:1443-5.
10 Laufer, L.R. et al. "Effect of Clonidine on Hot Flashes in Post-Menopausal Women." *Obstetrics & Gynecology.* 1982. 60:583-6.

against osteoporosis or cardiovascular symptoms.

Bellergal® has some unpleasant side effects. It may help those who can't take estrogen to get over the most severe vasomotor symptoms (hot flashes, insomnia, nervousness). It will not protect against osteoporosis or cardiovascular symptoms.

Some women feel acupuncture is helpful in controlling menopausal symptoms. Reliable studies have not been reported. More investigation is necessary before it can be recommended.

- *Because of breast cancer when I was 38, I am not supposed to take ERT. As part of my treatment, my ovaries were removed. The menopausal symptoms have been rough, but the most-severe symptom has been my inability to sleep. Isn't there anything I can do to get my sleep at night?*

Although over-the-counter medicines are not very strong, they are at least not addictive, so you might give them a try.

Many antihistamines have a side effect of making you sleepy, so you may want to try these. One advantage of these medicines is it is difficult to overdose with them. The disadvantage is they often produce drowsiness that may linger into the daytime. You should not drive after taking them. Never take these medications along with alcohol because the combined effect could produce symptoms of overdose.

Alcohol itself may produce drowsiness and help sleep, but it is also easy to become alcohol-dependent.

For many women, a low-dose antidepressant can produce a normal night's sleep and should not cause drug dependency.

- *My chief problem with menopause has been the wide mood swings which at first were relieved by ERT. But now the moodiness is beginning again despite ERT.*

ERT relieves most of these mood changes. If they are persisting or becoming worse, check with your doctor to see if there are deeper problems of a psychiatric nature. If mild medications will not relieve these symptoms, your doctor may want consultation with a psychiatrist early, before the changes become too severe.

ERT relieves most symptoms related to low estrogen levels very well. But this may lead both patients and doctors to expect 100-percent relief from all symptoms—something that is *not* possible. For those few women for whom ERT does not spell relief, carefully supervised hypothalamic depressors like

Xanax® or antidepressant medications can do wonders. But these must never be taken without meticulous monitoring by your doctor.

- *I have heard of a false menopause. What is this?*

A false menopause, called *pseudo-menopause,* is usually a *temporary* menopause that occurs when alterations in hormone production occur that simulate those found in menopause.

Excessive dieting, improper dieting (fad-dieting), excessive weight loss, anorexia nervosa, high level of exercise such as marathoning or stress, (such as sudden death in the family), can all shut down hormone production and cause your menstrual periods to stop. Example: ballet dancers, Olympic participants and marathon runners often experience a loss of menstrual flow during their intensive training. Recovery is nearly always spontaneous when the causative experience is over.

In the course of these episodes, such women are also at risk of losing mineral from their bones and decreasing their bone mass, just as they are during menopause.

- *What is surgical menopause?*

This is an "induced" menopause caused by surgically removing your ovaries, whether your uterus is removed or not. See page 17 for a detailed discussion of surgical menopause.

- *Are symptoms of a surgical menopause more severe than symptoms of a so-called natural menopause?*

Symptoms of a surgical menopause may be more severe because the loss of estrogen is sudden. In a spontaneous menopause you may "coast" into a menopause with a gradual loss of estrogen so slight that you scarcely notice any symptoms. However, the symptoms of both spontaneous and surgical menopause should respond readily to estrogen-replacement therapy (ERT).

- *Do menopausal women have more emotional problems than other women? In other words, are menopausal women inclined to be emotionally more unstable?*

No, menopausal women don't usually have more problems than non-menopausal women. It is important they be well informed and know what to expect. Menopause is not, and does not have to be, a time of ill health or emotional instability.

If you are knowledgeable and realize menopause is just as normal as the menarche (beginning of menstrual periods), there is no reason why you should not enjoy even better health than ever. Relief from menstrual periods, as well as freedom from the fear of pregnancy, can herald the beginning of a new life, a life of good health and well-being.

Menopause and the years following it can be a time of excitement and fulfillment, aided by a steady hand of maturity that will help you cope with whatever lies ahead.

- *How valuable are vaginal smears in diagnosing menopause? In other words, can my doctor help me know when I am going through menopause by taking a vaginal smear?*

A vaginal smear obtains a cell sample from the walls of the upper third of your vagina. By examining these cells, your doctor can get an idea how much estrogen there is in your vaginal tissues. Although vaginal cells are slow to respond to estrogen (even by as much as 3 months) a smear may be helpful.

Vaginal smears provide a useful guideline as to whether you require estrogen treatment. Another criterion is the presence of menopausal symptoms.

Another more-accurate measure of menopause is a blood test in which the FSH (follicle-stimulating hormone) is measured. Frequently, doctors combine vaginal smears with an FSH blood test to determine your hormone level and decide whether you require hormone treatment.

If you have had your uterus removed (simple hysterectomy) but still have your ovaries, your doctor can determine how well they are functioning by an FSH blood test or an estradiol blood level test to measure estrogen.

- *Does removal of one ovary hasten the onset of menopause?*

No. In general, if 80 percent of the follicles in both ovaries are removed, your reproductive life might be shortened, but your ovaries and your fertility show remarkable tenacity.

- *Are there any other factors that cause an earlier menopause?*

Infection, radiation (either X-ray or radium), chemotherapy and even smoking may shorten your menstrual life. Apparently some of the 3,000 compounds in cigarette smoke destroy oocytes (potential eggs) in your ovaries and shorten your menstrual life by about 2 years regardless of the amount you smoke. Also, exposure to other people's smoke can have a similar effect.[11]

- *Do women nowadays undergo menopause at a later age than they used to?*

Some studies indicate the age of menopause is slightly older now. In general, it has been around age 50 for many centuries. This is despite the fact women now are living much longer.

- *What other functions does estrogen perform besides causing menopause when it is not present?*

Estrogen has many functions. Beginning at adolescence, estrogen is the hormone that gradually transforms you from a girl into a mature woman. It causes fat to be deposited in the proper amounts in the proper places to give you those graceful, rounded, typically female contours. Estrogen also causes your breasts to develop.

When estrogen production ceases, some of these processes take place in reverse. As fat is lost from beneath your skin, you develop wrinkles. Your breasts lose their contour by losing fatty tissues.

Your hair becomes somewhat coarser and thinner, especially over your pubis and under your arms. You may get more facial hair. Other symptoms appear, letting you know your estrogen production is beginning to wane.

On the happier side, this same estrogen can be supplied artificially and effectively, see Chapter 12. While there are many functions of estrogen and many symptoms appear when it is no longer produced. As you will read, we can do some remarkable things for you to relieve these symptoms.

11 Everson, R.B. "Effect of Passive Exposure to Smoking on Age at Menopause." *British Medical Journal.* 1986. 299:792.

2

Surgical Menopause

Surgical menopause is removal of the ovaries during a surgical procedure. This stops the production of all hormones normally produced by the ovary, such as estrogen and progesterone.

Regardless of age at the time of surgery, removal of the ovaries prior to menopause places a woman at sudden and abrupt risk for all the symptoms and physical changes seen with a natural or spontaneous menopause. A surgical menopause places younger women at increased risk for cardiovascular disease earlier in life. And, there's the risk of progressive loss of bone mass unless they receive immediate ERT (estrogen-replacement therapy) following surgery. ERT prevents the abrupt appearance of these symptoms due to sudden loss of estrogen when the ovaries are removed.

- *Do you mean a hysterectomy does not put me through menopause?*

No. Hysterectomy means removal of your uterus. Removal of your uterus (hysterectomy) ends your menstrual periods and will prevent you from becoming pregnant. But it will not put you through menopause. It is your *ovaries* that control menopause.

A hysterectomy should put an end to your menstrual cramps, but you may still have some discomfort when you ovulate, called *mittelschmerz*, when an egg is released from your ovary.

- *What if my ovaries are removed and not my uterus? Will I go through menopause?*

Yes. With the removal of the ovaries you will go into immediate menopause. You may still have your uterus, but you will not have menstrual periods because menstrual flow is dependent upon your ovaries. You will also not conceive because without your ovaries, there are no eggs to be fertilized. You may develop hot flashes and other symptoms of menopause if your ovaries are removed, whether or not your uterus has been removed.

However, if you take replacement estrogen-progestogen, you may resume menstrual periods. But you will not be able to conceive because there are no ovaries to produce eggs.

- *Is my menopause likely to be more severe if my ovaries are removed surgically?*

Not necessarily. When your ovaries are removed, the secretion of estrogen is withdrawn suddenly. A spontaneous menopause is normally due to a gradual decline in the number of eggs in your ovaries, which in turn produces a gradual fall in the production of estrogen.

If you are immediately placed upon artificial hormones (estrogen and progestogen or ERT) after surgical removal of your ovaries, you may not notice any symptoms of menopause.

We have found women in the perimenopausal period (age 40 to 50) have been gradually adjusting to decreasing levels of estrogen and therefore accept surgical loss of their ovaries more easily. By contrast, women in their 20s and 30s have to adjust to the loss of a higher estrogen level and could have more severe symptoms following surgical menopause unless immediately placed on ERT.

- *What happens if only one ovary is removed surgically?*

Usually nothing. One ovary can produce enough estrogen to meet your needs. When both ovaries, or one plus most of the remaining ovary are removed, there may be a noticeable lack of estrogen.

We have seen instances in which pregnancy occurs when only a tiny piece of one ovary is left at surgery. There were no symptoms of the change (menopause) at all. Nature's marvelous recuperative ability seems to rise to the occasion when we least expect it.

- *Doesn't hysterectomy mean removing the ovaries too?*

No. Hysterectomy means only the removal of the uterus and cervix. Total abdominal hysterectomy means the removal of the

༄   ༄   ༄

Some hospitals and most insurance companies require consultation (a second opinion) before your doctor can perform a hysterectomy.

uterus and cervix through an incision on the abdomen.

Although your ovaries, if diseased, are removed along with the uterus, normal ovaries are usually left in place when a woman is under age 45. At 45, the question of removing the ovaries becomes a possibility but not an automatic procedure. Your ovaries then have 3 to 8 years of function left. If they are removed, you will have to take hormones to prevent osteoporosis and to relieve symptoms of menopause.

Removing the ovaries is called *oophorectomy.*

- *Then why remove the ovaries if they are normal?*

Although cancer of the ovary is not common, it does occur. According to the American Cancer Society (1990), it causes an estimated 20,500 deaths each year in the United States. Less than 1 out of 70 women will develop cancer of the ovary in a lifetime. One of the reasons for poor cure statistics in cancer of the ovary is it usually does not cause symptoms until it has progressed too far to be cured.

Typically, cancer of the ovary is a "silent" disease. It seldom produces bleeding or pain until far advanced. The usual way cancer of the ovary is diagnosed is by pelvic examination, something too many women neglect to have on a regular basis.

Many hysterectomies are done through the vagina, which is an excellent method of removal. But it is more difficult to remove the ovaries through a vaginal approach, so the tendency is to leave them in place.

- *Should I request my doctor remove my ovaries when he removes my uterus, even if they are normal?*

Much depends upon your age. If you are under 45, we advise you to leave your ovaries, assuming they are normal. They have many years of function left in them. (See next question.)

After 45, you should have your ovaries removed prophylactically to avoid the threat of cancer. Only a few years of function are left in them anyway. Beyond 50, we strongly suggest your ovaries be removed at the time of a hysterectomy, even if they are normal.

- *What are the disadvantages of having my ovaries removed if I am having the uterus removed anyway?*

Removal of your ovaries means sudden onset of menopause with its uncomfortable symptoms, for which you would require

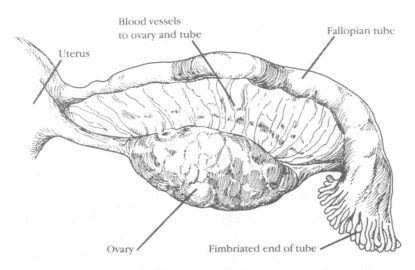

Blood vessels
to ovary and tube

Fallopian tube

Uterus

Ovary

Fimbriated end of tube

Because the ovary and fallopian tube share a blood supply, they are usually removed together during surgery. This is true unless there is some special reason to remove one and leave the other.

hormonal treatment if there are no medical reasons not to do so. It also means calcium loss from your bones (osteoporosis with possible fractures) will be accelerated unless you take estrogen along with calcium.

- *What happens to the eggs that are released from the ovaries if I have my uterus removed, yet leave the ovaries?*

Eggs continue to be released from your ovaries at least one each month until such time as you go through menopause. These eggs are simply absorbed in the abdominal cavity. Remember that ova are microscopic in size.

You may continue to have discomfort when you ovulate, called *mittelschmerz*, especially if you've had discomfort in the past.

- *If I have my uterus removed and it is found to be cancerous, yet my ovaries have been left, what then?*

If you have a hysterectomy in which cancer is found and your ovaries have not been removed, then your ovaries would have to be removed in another operation. This could vary according to the type of cancer and its extent. Yes, this means an extra operation if it proves necessary.

- *Will X-ray treatments harm my ovaries?*

It depends upon what kind of treatments, how many and what area of your body is treated. X-ray may not only harm, it may obliterate the function of your ovaries. In some instances, this is unavoidable and even desirable. If you are younger and not menopausal, an effort will be made to shield your ovaries from the X-ray.

- *Will chemotherapy cause menopause?*

In some instances, yes. There are many different types of chemotherapy. It also depends on the dosage that is given and for how long. Chemotherapy given to treat cancer of the breast will cause premature menopause in women younger than 40. This is acceptable because survival is the important goal of treatment.

In the case of hydatidiform mole (cystic degeneration of cells of the placenta), the risk of cancer and the threat to life is considerably less. If you want more children, less chemotherapy may be given to preserve your ability to conceive.

- *Does a hysterectomy in which my ovaries are left in place cause me to go through menopause earlier than normal?*

Menopause may occur a few years earlier, possibly due to some interference with the blood supply to the ovaries. Many women do not notice any menopausal symptoms after a simple hysterectomy until the usual time a spontaneous menopause occurs.

I am scheduled to have a hysterectomy in which the doctor says he will also remove my ovaries. I am 45 years old. He has not mentioned the fallopian tubes. What happens to them?

Because they share blood supply with your ovaries, the fallopian tubes are simply removed along with the ovaries. They serve no purpose after removal of your ovaries and uterus.

- *From the standpoint of sexual response is there any advantage to leaving one ovary and removing the other when a hysterectomy is done after the age of 45?*

No. One ovary secretes sufficient estrogen to prevent menopause, but it still leaves the possibility of cancer. Sexual response should be unaffected in either event.

ᴣ᰿   ᴣ᰿   ᴣ᰿

A hysterectomy puts a permanent end to your childbearing.

- *Will I have to take more hormones after my hysterectomy than if I had just gone through normal menopause? I am 43 years old.*

We have found patients of your age who have a hysterectomy with removal of the ovaries do not require any more hormones to relieve their symptoms than those women who go through menopause naturally. Sometimes it seems the symptoms are easier to control after a hysterectomy because there is no uterus from which the hormones can cause you to bleed.

There is another consideration, however. A hysterectomy plus removal of your ovaries plunges you into sudden menopause (sudden loss of estrogen). A spontaneous menopause is more likely to ease you into a gradual withdrawal of estrogen. Our experience has been that women who have premature menopause through surgery may require more "fine tuning," more adjusting and more time to find just the right dose of estrogen.

3

Cancer & Menopause

Cancer is sure to touch the life of everyone in some way. Yet, few even know what it is. As a matter of fact, doctors can only describe its characteristics.

Cancer is not really one disease, but a series of diseases sharing certain characteristics we will discuss later. First, let's describe a normal cell, so you can better understand what a cancer cell is.

A normal cell has a nucleus in its center surrounded by material known as *cytoplasm*. A normal cell will not change from one type of cell into another. For example, a skin cell remains a skin cell and a muscle cell remains a muscle cell. All healthy, normal cells work together for the good of your body and will do nothing to harm your body or other cells of your body.

By contrast, a cancer cell refuses to abide by the rules. It changes its appearance and behavior in the following ways:

1. Its nucleus becomes larger and darker in color.
2. Material inside nucleus becomes jumbled and disorganized.
3. Cell becomes irregular in shape.
4. Cancer cells no longer stay in normal formation but begin to pile up on each other.
5. Cancer cells rob nourishment from other cells, growing and reproducing much faster than other cells.
6. Cancer cells crowd, push and compress normal cells that get in their way, gradually causing death of normal cells by starvation and suffocation.
7. Finally, the cancer cells "take over" the entire area as they crowd out all normal cells. This is called *in situ cancer*— it is limited to that area and has not yet begun to spread.

Cancer cells have the following common characteristics:

1. They grow fast enough to crowd out normal tissue that gets in their way.

2. They no longer look or act like the original tissue from which they came.
3. They no longer serve the body, but work against it.
4. They will eventually cause death if they are not removed or killed by some method.

Fortunately we have methods to kill some cancers and we know enough to prevent the development of many others.

- *How does cancer spread?*

As cancer cells continue to grow and multiply at rapid speed, they break through natural barriers and begin to spread to adjacent tissues. At first this spread may be confined to just one organ. But soon the cancer breaks through the capsule of the organ and spreads to surrounding organs. This is called *extension* or *local spread* of the cancer.

In the process of spreading, the cancer may break through the walls of blood vessels or lymph channels and be carried to lymph glands or to other organs in the body. This is called *distant spread* or *metastasis.*

- *Why does cancer seem to attack or localize in certain organs more than others?*

Because cancer cells are growing and multiplying rapidly, they have a tremendous need for oxygen and a voracious appetite for nourishment. Consequently they seek out those organs with the richest blood supply—liver, brain, bone marrow and lungs. They become "trapped" in the lymph nodes because the body directs most of its enemies to these glands in hopes they can be overcome. The same process occurs with infection and causes swollen glands at the time of a sore throat, for instance.

- *What causes cancer?*

We know that:

1. Some leukemias (cancer of white blood cells) may be associated with certain types of radiation.
2. Some skin cancers are caused by the sun's rays.
3. Some cancers are caused by chemicals and toxins in our environment.
4. Some cancers, such as cancers of the cervix, are associated with viruses.
5. Many lung cancers are linked to cigarette smoking.

6. Some cancers, such as cancer of the endometrium, may be linked to estrogen when it is given without progestogen.

7. Some cancers are caused by diet.

We do not know the cause of most cancers.

- *Is cancer inherited?*

There are certain kinds of cancer in which a tendency or proneness seems to be inherited. For instance, if your mother or your sister has had cancer of the breast, there is a 2 to 3 times greater chance of your developing cancer of the breast. Such facts lead us to believe that some hereditary factor may be involved.

- *Am I more likely to develop any kind of cancer during menopause?*

As you grow older, your chances of developing most cancers seem to increase but not just because of menopause.

Cancer of the Uterus

- *How common is cancer of the uterus?*

According to 1990 statistics from the American Cancer Society (1990), most of the 46,500 cancers of the uterus that occur in women each year in the United States can be divided into 33,000 cancers of the endometrium (inner lining of the uterus) and 13,500 cancers of the cervix.

- *What is the difference between cancer of the cervix and cancer of the uterus?*

As you see in the illustration, the uterus consists of two principal parts: the corpus (body) and the cervix (neck). When we speak of cancer of the uterus, we usually mean cancer of the corpus. Specifically, this is cancer of the uterine-cavity lining, called endometrium or *endometrial cancer.*

Cancer of the neck of the uterus usually involves the opening of the cervix, referred to as *cancer of the cervix.* Endometrial and cervical cancers involve different types of cells. They therefore act very differently in nearly every respect and must be treated as separate diseases, despite the fact both occur in the uterus.

- *How does a Pap smear detect cancer? Which type of cancer does it detect?*

A Pap smear is taken from the opening of the cervix.The cervix

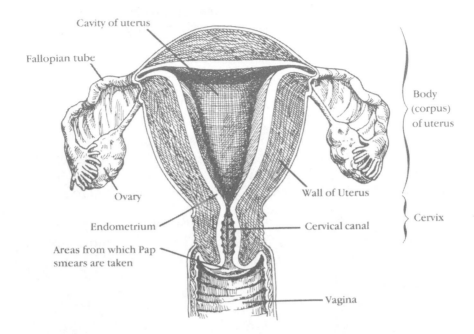

Front view of female internal organs.

is the "neck" of the uterus and the part of the uterus that protrudes into the vagina. If you reach a finger into your vagina and
touch the tip of your cervix, it feels about the consistency of your
nose. When you become pregnant, the cervix softens and feels
similar to your lips when pursed to whistle. Cancer is most likely
to develop in this opening of the cervix. A Pap smear "samples"
cells from this area.

• *My doctor told me not to take a vaginal douche for a day or two before
I come for my Pap smear. Why?*

A Pap smear samples cells taken from the opening of the cervix.
If you douche, you are likely to wash out most of the cells your
doctor wants to sample in the Pap smear.

A tiny, soft brush obtains a sample that is "rolled" onto a slide
for analysis. The procedure is painless.

• *What is the relationship of herpes infection to cancer of the cervix?*

Your chance of developing cancer of the cervix is increased as
much as 8 times if you have genital herpes. Additional studies
are also incriminating genitourinary warts.

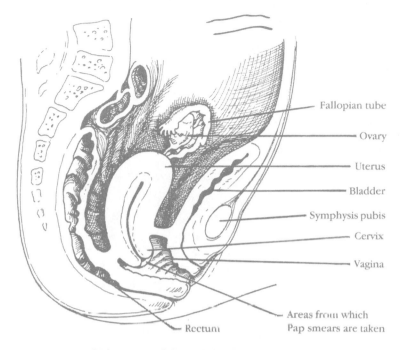

Side view of female internal organs.

We don't know if there is something in sperm that also influences cancer of the cervix. It has been shown that women who begin intercourse at a young age and have multiple sex partners are more likely to develop cancer of the cervix. This why we recommend women have a Pap smear soon after their first sexual encounter and repeat Pap smears at yearly intervals thereafter.

Some physicians feel a yearly Pap smear is unnecessary. According to a reliable study of cancer of the cervix during 1977 through 1979 by the Kaiser Foundation, about 20 percent of the patients with cancer of the cervix had shown two *negative* Pap smears within 3 years of the diagnosis of this cancer.

Not to discredit the accuracy nor the value of the Pap smear, its quoted false-negative rate varies from 2.6 percent to 26 percent. An annual Pap smear improves the chance of detecting abnormal cells that may develop.

- *How common is cancer of the cervix?*

About 2 percent of women past 40 will develop cancer of the cervix. This cancer is an almost-preventable disease. Cervical dysplasia can progress to cancer in 3 to 7 years. A regular Pap smear helps detect these changes early.

The American Cancer Society says that if you have 2 successive negative Pap smears you need have them only every 3 to 5 years until 65. After 65 you can discontinue having them. The American College of Obstetricians and Gynecologists recommends a *yearly* Pap smear. This brings you into the doctor's office more often. Not only cancer of the cervix but other conditions can be discovered and treated earlier.

- *What are my chances for cure if I develop cancer of the cervix?*

  Cancer of the cervix is treatable and curable if diagnosed early enough. Early diagnosis can be assured by regular Pap smears. A positive diagnosis by smear must be confirmed by biopsy. Treatment of cancer of the cervix is by surgery, radiation or a combination of these methods. If regular Pap smears could somehow be taken, death due to cancer of the cervix could almost be eliminated.

- *Why are certain people more likely to develop cancer of the cervix?*

  Cancer of the cervix is more common in:

  1. Those who are sexually active from their mid-teens.
  2. Those who have multiple sex partners.
  3. Those who have genital herpes.
  4. Those in the lower socioeconomic groups.
  5. Those who have human papilloma viruses (venereal warts) manifested as cauliflower-like growths on the genitals.
  6. Those whose sex partners are uncircumcised.
  7. Those who smoke.

- *How long does it take for a suspicious lesion on the cervix to develop into a definite cancer?*

  This question is difficult to answer. According to DiSaia and Creasman (1984), it takes about 4.5 years for a smear to change from normal to an *in situ* cancer (earliest definite cancer before any spread). It is not possible to predict which patients will remain with this very early cancer and which will have cancer that progresses to the invasive stage and/or within what time frame.

  At least we know cancer of the cervix is usually a slow-growing cancer. Early cancers which are still in the treatable and curable

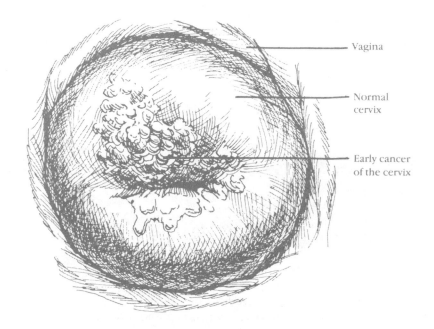

Early cancer of the cervix.

stage can be detected through a Pap smear.

- *Do I need to have a Pap smear if I am past menopause?*

There is some controversy over this. In general, a Pap smear on an annual basis is recommended primarily because it will cause you to have an annual physical examination, including a pelvic examination. In our own practices we've uncovered countless other conditions that otherwise would have remained undiagnosed and untreated.

Ovarian tumors, hernias, melanomas (cancerous moles), diabetes, hypertension, hemorrhoids severe enough to warrant surgery, breast masses, cervicitis and sexually transmitted diseases are just a few of the conditions that turned up during the annual visit for a Pap smear.

Although cancer of the cervix after age 65 is unlikely, we have these patients return for an annual Pap smear. It brings them in for a regular check-up in which some of the above conditions are uncovered.

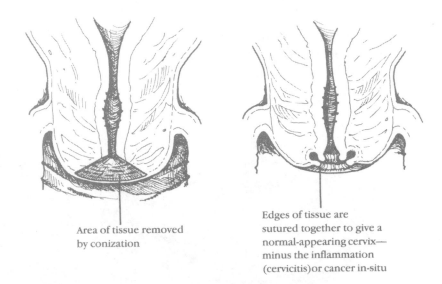

Area of tissue removed
by conization

Edges of tissue are
sutured together to give a
normal-appearing cervix—
minus the inflammation
(cervicitis)or cancer in-situ

*This is the area of tissue removed by conization. Tissue edges
are stitched together to give a normal-appearing cervix.*

- *Do I need a Pap smear if I have had my uterus removed?*

  On rare occasions, a cancer of the vagina may be diagnosed by a
  Pap smear. But this disease is so uncommon that a Pap smear *only*
  for this purpose seems unwarranted. However, cells from your
  vaginal wall are also evaluated for estrogen content. This information is helpful in determining the course of estrogen-replacement therapy.

  Occasionally, at the time hysterectomy is performed, a small
  piece of cervical tissue is inadvertently left in the vagina. This
  could become malignant. The best reason for an annual visit
  remains: To have a check-up by your doctor.

- *Does a Pap smear diagnose other cancers besides cancer of the cervix?*

  Once in a while cancer of the endometrium is diagnosed by a Pap
  smear. The Pap smear is designed primarily to examine the cells
  from your cervix. A Pap smear should certainly not be relied
  upon to diagnose cancer of the endometrium.

- *What is a cervical biopsy and how is it performed?*

  If you have an abnormal Pap smear or an abnormal-appearing
  cervix, a sample of tissue is taken from the cervix and examined
  under the microscope. This is called a *biopsy* of the cervix. A Pap

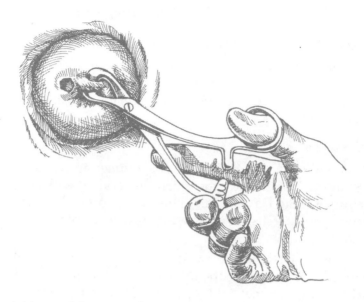

A punch biopsy of the cervix may be used to diagnose or confirm cancer of the cervix.

smear can suggest cancer of the cervix, but a positive diagnosis depends upon a cervical biopsy.

A painful sensation in your cervix may come from dilating its opening. Your doctor may cut, burn (cauterize) or stitch your cervix without your feeling any discomfort. No anesthetic is necessary for a cervical biopsy. This procedure can be carried out in your doctor's office. A biopsy may be taken from suspicious areas on the cervix as identified under the colposcope, a microscope used specifically to view the tissues of your vulva, vagina and cervix.

If the smear suggests a cancer of tissue that lies deeper in the cervical canal or if your doctor requires a more adequate specimen for biopsy, he will remove a cone of tissue from your cervix. This is called *conization* of the cervix. See illustration.

Cancer of the Endometrium

- *How common is cancer of the endometrium?*

Endometrial cancer is the most common malignancy seen in the female pelvis today. The American Cancer Society estimated that more than 33,000 women developed uterine cancer in 1990 in the United States.

- *What is a D&C?*

D&C actually stands for *Dilation & Curettage,* in which the cervix is first dilated (stretched), the uterus is scraped with a semisharp instrument called a *curette.* This same procedure is used to remove residual tissue following most spontaneous miscarriages.

In midlife, a D&C is the most thorough method to diagnose cancer of the lining of the uterus when you have abnormal bleeding. An endometrial biopsy can first be performed in your doctor's office often under a paracervical (local) block anesthesia.

- *What is a clinical or medical D&C?*

By administering female sex hormones in a cyclic fashion, then withdrawing them, a so-called *clinical D&C* is accomplished in which the endometrial tissue is sloughed off. Although this may remove the lining, it does not provide tissue for microscopic diagnosis and respective treatment.

A clinical D&C is helpful in treating recurrent bleeding after you have had a D&C to rule out cancer. Sometimes it cures bleeding which occurs when your hormones are not functioning as they should.

- *What is an endometrial biopsy?*

An endometrial biopsy is a sampling of tissue from the inner lining of the uterine cavity. It is like a miniature D&C.

Endometrial biopsies are reliable in about 90 percent of patients in diagnosing cancer of the inner lining of the uterus (DiSaia & Creasman, 1984). The definitive diagnosis and staging (determines how extensive and fast-growing it is) of endometrial cancer is made by a fractional D&C. In a fractional D&C, the endometrial tissue as well as the tissue from the cervical canal is completely sampled to determine the extension of the cancer.

- *Are certain women more likely to develop cancer of the endometrium?*

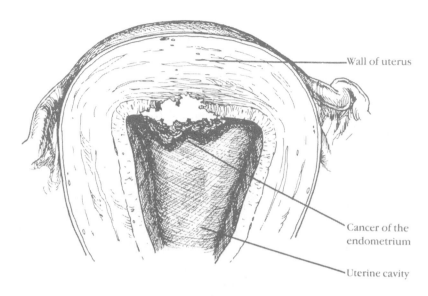

Cancer of the endometrium is cancer of the lining of the uterine cavity. It is commonly called cancer of the uterus.

Cancer of the endometrium is more common in women whose ovaries secrete too much estrogen. Women who do not ovulate or those who have what we call *dysfunctional* (abnormal or irregular) uterine bleeding are also more likely to develop endometrial cancer. Because these women usually have difficulty conceiving, this type of cancer is more common in those who have had no children.

Cancer of the endometrium is also more common in those women who have high blood pressure, diabetes, or who are obese.

Risk of Endometrial Cancer		
Therapy Group	Patient Years of Observation	Incidence of Endometrial Cancer (per 100,000)
Estrogen + Progesterone Users	11,895	68.1
Estrogen Users Not Taking Progesterone	15,605	410.8
Untreated Women	5,285	258.1
Adapted from R. D. Gambrell, Jr., Physician and Patient, 1983:1		

- *Tell me, does estrogen cause cancer of the uterus?*

  Estrogen does *not* cause cancer of the uterus if it is taken properly, which means progestogen is given for 12 to 13 days each month along with the estrogen. In fact, ERT (estrogen-replacement therapy) including progestogen is believed to protect against development of cancer of the uterus.

  If taken alone, estrogen may cause the lining of your uterus to build up (endometrial hyperplasia), a precancerous condition.

- *What are the common signs of cancer of the endometrium?*

  The most common sign of cancer of the endometrium is abnormal uterine bleeding. Before menopause this may appear as bleeding (spotting) between your menstrual periods or irregular periods. Endometrial cancer may also cause heavier and longer bleeding than normal. Certainly if you have any bleeding after menopause, you should check immediately with your physician who can determine the cause of the bleeding and treat you accordingly. Any bleeding, spotting or blood staining after menopause should be considered a sign of cancer until proved otherwise.

- *How effective is treatment for cancer of the endometrium?*

  Treatment of cancer of the endometrium depends mostly upon how advanced the cancer is. The specific type of cancer is also important because some cancers grow faster and spread sooner than others. Some cancers are more sensitive to irradiation and chemotherapy.

  Surgery, radium, chemotherapy or any combination of these methods may be used to treat cancer of the endometrium. The outlook for endometrial cancer is excellent if the diagnosis is made fairly early, with 5-year-survival rates of up to 95 percent.

- *I am 48. My menstrual periods are very irregular. Some last for 2 weeks. My friends tell me this is normal for menopause and if I will just be patient for a few months, it will be over.*

  Your friends are wrong. While the irregular bleeding is probably due to the adjustment of your body to the decreasing estrogen, it could also be an early sign of endometrial hyperplasia or even cancer of the uterus. Why take a chance when this type of cancer is so easy to treat and cure if detected early?

  See your doctor if your menstrual periods are irregular, heavier than normal, prolonged or even if you skip them. It will help to

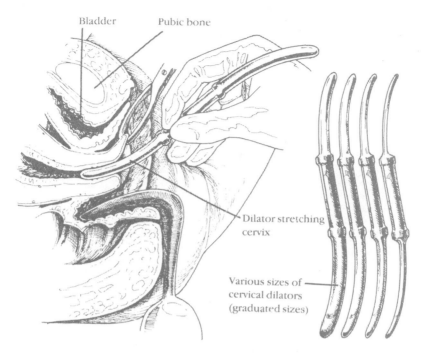

Dilation of the cervix. Before the uterine cavity can be scraped, the cervix must be dilated so instruments can enter.

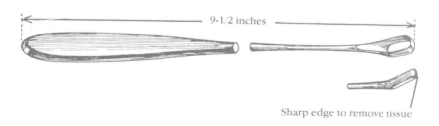

A sharp curette is the instrument used to scrape the lining of the uterus in a D&C.

put your mind at ease.

- *Is spotting ever considered normal during menopause?*

Spotting is common during menopause because of decreasing estrogen production by the ovaries. When ovulation fails to occur because of the diminishing number of ova, the lining in your uterus continues to thicken until it reaches the point where it

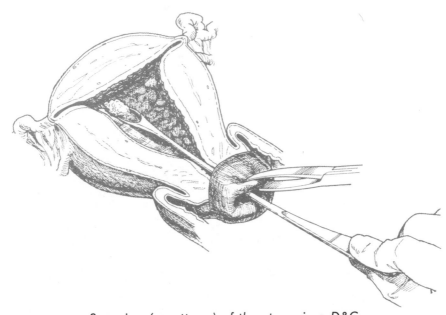

Scraping (curettage) of the uterus in a D&C.

begins to fragment. At this point, irregular and often unpredictable bleeding occurs.

Although this type of bleeding is common at menopause, it cannot be taken for granted or ignored. Because endometrial cancer is common at this age, a thorough endometrial biopsy or—if necessary—a D&C must be performed to rule out cancer. However, the usual cause of the bleeding is endometrial hyperplasia (excessive thickening of the lining of the uterus).

• *How would I know if I had the precancerous condition of the lining of the uterus called* endometrial hyperplasia?

It is possible to develop endometrial hyperplasia even though you are not taking estrogen. When your body does not produce progesterone to complete the process of a menstrual cycle with sloughing off of the lining of the uterus, hyperplasia results.

The most common symptoms of endometrial hyperplasia are irregular, prolonged or heavy bleeding. *Any* abnormal bleeding in conjunction with or following menopause should be reported to your doctor immediately. Keep in mind there are also other causes of abnormal bleeding at this or any age.

A Pap smear is not sufficient to determine the cause of abnormal

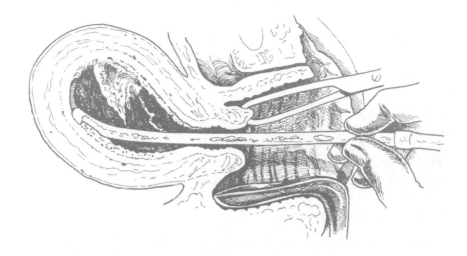

Vacutage uses suction to remove the contents, including the lining of the uterus. Most often it is used for abortion, but also occasionally for diagnosis of the inner lining of the uterus.

bleeding. An endometrial biopsy (sampling) is usually necessary. A D&C may also be done to rule out the possibility of cancer.

- *Would you say endometrial hyperplasia and cancer of the endometrium are preventable?*

Almost. There are always exceptions to rules. If endometrial cancer does develop, it can and should be diagnosed early and can usually be treated successfully. It has a 95-percent 5-year-cure rate.

Because we recommend ERT for nearly every woman after menopause, we also recommend that every woman have what we call a *progesterone challenge,* see page 169, when she has stopped bleeding for several months. If she bleeds following this test, she should have an endometrial biopsy to rule out endometrial hyperplasia or cancer of the endometrium. Following a negative biopsy she may then be placed on ERT.

If every woman placed on ERT after menopause were followed conscientiously as indicated above, endometrial hyperplasia and cancer of the endometrium would be practically nonexistent.

- *If ERT does not cause cancer, why is it not recommended for postmenopausal women who have had cancer of the breast or cancer of the uterus?*

Estrogen-replacement therapy is not given to women who have had estrogen-related cancer of the breast or uterus because estrogen could stimulate the growth of any residual cancer that was not cured by the treatment. Estrogen alone does not seem to be a carcinogen (cancer causer). There is some controversy as to the type of estrogen used (natural versus synthetic), the use of progestogen and other risk factors such as family history, smoking, high-fat diet, alcohol use, etc. that may increase the risk of developing breast cancer for those women using estrogen longer than 15 years. Estrogen will not cause uterine cancer if given along with a progestogen.

- *I had endometrial cancer 5 years ago and was successfully treated. I am still having severe hot flashes and dryness of the vagina with painful intercourse. Can I safely take ERT now?*

Check with your doctor. It will depend upon the kind of cancer, the degree of involvement of the uterus and the amount of spread. If you are not a candidate for estrogen, you may find progestogen alone will be helpful in relieving your flashes. Try Replens®, a long-lasting vaginal moisturizer or a water-soluble lubricating jelly such as H-R®, K-Y® or Lubafax® to help relieve your dryness and dyspareunia (painful intercourse).

- *How do I know when my uterine bleeding is too much?*

We have already mentioned that bleeding between menstrual periods must be checked out by endometrial biopsy or D&C, but so-called heavy bleeding is a relative thing. In general, *any* change in your menstrual periods warrants checking with your physician.

If your menstrual periods have always been light and suddenly become heavy, go for a checkup. If your periods are longer or heavier than normal, check with your doctor. She will know if an endometrial biopsy or a D&C is necessary.

- *Are fibroid tumors ever cancerous?*

Yes, but rarely. It is estimated that less than 2 percent of fibroid tumors ever become malignant. If these common tumors become large enough they cause pressure on your bladder or other pelvic organs; if they cause abnormal bleeding (usually heavy); if they

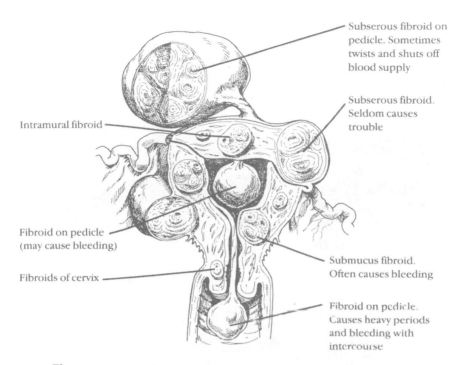

Subserous fibroid on pedicle. Sometimes twists and shuts off blood supply

Subserous fibroid. Seldom causes trouble

Intramural fibroid

Fibroid on pedicle (may cause bleeding)

Fibroids of cervix

Submucus fibroid. Often causes bleeding

Fibroid on pedicle. Causes heavy periods and bleeding with intercourse

There are many locations for fibroid tumors of the uterus.
Size and location often determine symptoms.

cause pain; or if they are preventing pregnancy, surgical removal may be necessary.

About 40 percent of women have fibroid tumors by the time they reach menopause, but only 10 percent or less will have sufficient symptoms to warrant surgery.

- *Is it ever possible to remove only the fibroid tumor and leave my uterus?*

Yes, this is called a *myomectomy*. If you have symptoms severe enough to demand surgery, it is better to have a hysterectomy unless you desire more children.

- *My doctor said I had an enlarged uterus, and it has worried me ever since. He did not suggest surgery. What does this mean?*

Pregnancy often leaves the uterus larger than it was before the pregnancy began. Your uterus may enlarge a little more with each child. Unless your uterus has enlarged enough to make your doctor suspicious of a tumor, you do not need to worry about normal enlargement after having children.

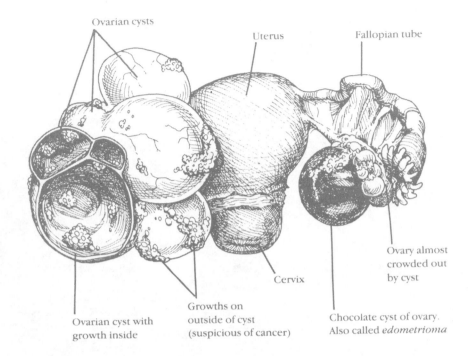

Ovarian cysts

Uterus

Fallopian tube

Ovary almost
crowded out
by cyst

Cervix

Ovarian cyst with
growth inside

Growths on
outside of cyst
(suspicious of cancer)

Chocolate cyst of ovary.
Also called *edometrioma*

This composite shows an endometrial cyst (chocolate cyst) on one side and many cysts on the other side, with growths on the inside and outside of the cyst.

- *I do not want any more children. Wouldn't it be better to have my uterus removed, so I wouldn't have to worry about cancer or pregnancy?*

  Hysterectomy is a major operation and entails some risks and complications. If fertility is a big concern, you might want to consider tubal ligation (tying tubes) for sterilization. It is a simple procedure with minimal risk.

  Because of the risk that accompanies hysterectomy, this operation should not be performed only to avoid cancer or just for sterilization.

- *My doctor told me the tissues (uterus, tubes and ovaries) he removed were non-malignant. Does that mean absolutely I do not have cancer?*

  Yes, the terms *malignant* and *cancerous* are the same.

- *Can radiation (X-rays) cause menopause?*

  Yes. Radiation treatment in sufficient amount can cause your ovaries to atrophy (dry up) and fail to function, just as if they had been removed by surgery. Routine X-rays for diagnostic purposes should have no effect on ovarian function or menopause.

Cancer of the Ovary

- *How common is cancer of the ovary?*

  Cancer of the ovary is the fifth leading cause of cancer death in women, with about 20,500 lives lost each year in the United States. White women between 55 and 75 are more susceptible to cancer of the ovary. If you have surgery during your late 40s or 50s this may influence you to have your ovaries removed at the same time as a hysterectomy, even though they are normal.

- *Does the birth-control pill increase the risk of cancer of the ovary?*

  No. In fact, most recent studies indicate women who are taking birth-control pills have a 50 percent less chance of developing cancer of the ovary. Those who have taken them develop less ovarian cancer. They even have an improved prognosis if they do develop ovarian cancer.

- *You have mentioned that cancer of the ovary is a silent disease. Can't it be diagnosed by a routine sonogram?*

  Ultrasound cannot diagnose cancer. It can only show changes in the size, cystic or solid areas, or irregularities of the ovaries that make us suspicious of possible cancer.

- *What symptoms should I look for in cancer of the ovary?*

  Unfortunately there are no symptoms of early ovarian cancer. In general, you must wait until you have symptoms such as abdominal pain or pelvic discomfort or abnormal bleeding if you still have your uterus. Abdominal enlargement, pain or a mass in your abdomen are usually symptoms of advanced disease.

  Enlargement of your ovary is detected by a pelvic examination, ultrasound, or by laparoscopy, see pages 137–139.

&⁊ &⁊ &⁊

An enlarged abdomen is occasionally assumed to be due to pregnancy when it is really a tumor—and vice versa.

- *If I have abdominal pain, abnormal bleeding or an enlarged ovary, how can my doctor know if I have ovarian cancer?*

  If your doctor suspects enlargement of your ovary, ultrasound can help to differentiate an ovarian tumor from a mass in some other organ, such as the bowel. Any ovarian mass larger than 6 centimeters (2.4 inches) in diameter should be explored surgically to rule out cancer (DiSaia & Creasman, 1984).

  In some instances laparoscopy is helpful in distinguishing ovarian cysts from solid ovarian tumors.

- *What is the difference between laparotomy and laparoscopy?*

  Laparotomy is an ordinary incision into your abdominal cavity to perform whatever surgery is necessary. *Laparoscopy* involves making a 1/4-inch incision in the navel through which a pencil-size tube (laparoscope) with a series of mirrors and a light is inserted. This scope allows your doctor to inspect and biopsy your ovaries or other organs. See pages 137–139.

  Through a laparoscope your doctor can determine the type and size of pelvic mass and whether it has spread beyond the ovary. Laparoscopy is especially helpful if the entire question of a "pelvic mass" is uncertain.

- *What is the outlook for cancer of the ovary?*

  There are many types of cancer of the ovary. The treatment and outlook vary according to the type of cancer and the stage at which diagnosis is made.

  Cancer of the ovary characteristically causes few if any symptoms until it has spread. It is known as the "silent" cancer because of its usual lack of symptoms. This is one very important reason for having an *annual* physical exam.

- *Is it better to remove normal ovaries at the time of hysterectomy to avoid future cancer?*

  Because 80 percent or more of ovarian cancers are found in women past 50, the question arises as to prophylactic removal of ovaries in women who have a hysterectomy. If your ovaries are removed, you will likely have menopausal symptoms from then on. On the other hand, if your ovaries are not removed, they become a silent threat of cancer.

  After 50, everyone agrees the ovaries (even if normal) should be removed if a hysterectomy (removal of the uterus) is performed.

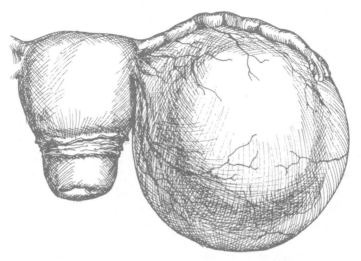

Benign (non-cancerous) cyst of the ovary.

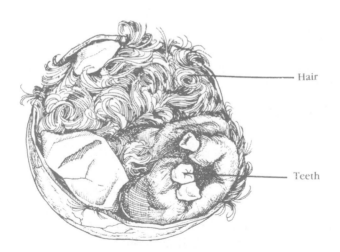

Hair

Teeth

A dermoid cyst is a benign cyst of the ovary that has various tissues in it.
It can become cancerous and is then called a teratoma.

Prior to this age there is some controversy. Some physicians feel ovaries should be removed after the age of 45 when a hysterectomy is performed. The decision should be left to the discretion and choice of the patient after the advantages and disadvantages have been explained.

If you want to have your ovaries removed, you must realize you will have to take estrogen to replace their function, but you then will not have to worry about "silent" ovarian cancers.

Cancer of the Breast

• *How common is cancer of the breast?*

Cancer of the breast will strike about 1 in 9 women during their lifetime. It accounts for 18 percent of cancer deaths in women (1990 statistics of the American Cancer Society). Until cancer of the lung took over recently, cancer of the breast was the most common cause of death in women. With increased smoking among women, lung cancer now accounts for 21 percent of cancer deaths in women.

• *Is there any way to increase early detection of cancer of the breast?*

According to DiSaia & Creasman (1984), over 70 percent of lumps in the breast are discovered by women themselves and not by their doctors. Certainly this reenforces the importance of breast self-examination. Every woman over age 20 should learn how to examine her own breasts. She should check them at least once a month, preferably right after her menstrual period, when all soreness and tender swelling are gone. Early detection can also be aided by screening mammography beginning at age 35.

• *Should I have a mammogram and when?*

Have your first (*baseline*) mammogram at age 35. If it is normal, have another at age 40, then every 2 years until 50 and every year thereafter.

With modern techniques, a mammogram subjects you to minimal radiation. Yet it can detect cancers too small to be felt by self-examination or even by your doctor. About 85 percent of breast cancers can be cured if detected early and before they spread.

• *How should I check my breasts for cancer?*

1. Check your breasts monthly, right after your menstrual period or by the calendar if your periods have stopped.

2. Examining your breasts while they are wet gives you a more accurate "feel." In the shower or tub you have an excellent opportunity to check yourself. You will soon come to know

yourself and your breasts. If something abnormal appears, you should be able to detect it readily.

3. Check yourself both in the upright position and while lying down. Gently roll the tissue in your right breast under the flat part of the fingers of your left hand in a circular motion. Check each segment of your breast. Check first while your arm is extended along your head. Then drop your arm to your side while you check for lumps in your armpit.

4. Repeat the same procedure in the opposite arm.

5. Following your bath or shower, lie down on the bed on your back and carefully repeat the process. Check each segment of each breast with the same circular motion while your breast is flattened out.

6. Stand in front of the mirror to see if you detect any bulging or puckering in either breast. Also check to see if there is any displacement of either nipple.

7. Have a baseline mammogram at age 35. A breast examination will be done each year by your physician as part of your annual physical examination.

- *My breasts are actually "lumpy," especially just before my menstrual period. What causes this?*

Fibrocystic disease is a condition in which your breasts have countless lumps in them. These lumps are more noticeable just before your menstrual period. The lumps in this most-common disease are rarely cancerous. Check with your doctor just in case. Let her decide whether they need to be biopsied.

Occasionally these lumps and repeated biopsies become so troublesome that the breast must be removed. The skin is left intact (a subcutaneous mastectomy) and a prosthesis is inserted. The prosthesis, by the way, may look better than the original.

- *Can a breast cyst be checked or treated other than by surgical removal?*

Yes. If aspiration (page 51) removes all of it, no further treatment is necessary. If a mass remains after aspiration, the mass can be biopsied with a special biopsy needle or it can be removed surgically.

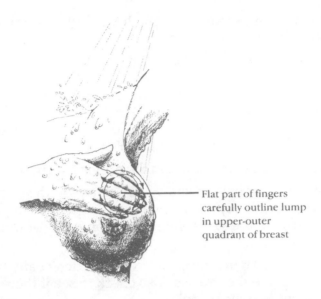

Flat part of fingers
carefully outline lump
in upper-outer
quadrant of breast

During a shower is a good time to check your breasts; touch is more sensitive when skin is wet. The most likely place for cancer is toward the armpit, in the upper, outer quadrant (quarter circle) of the breast.

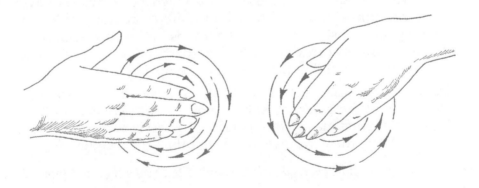

Rotation method of examining your breast for lumps. Use the flat part of your fingers to examine your breast, then reverse direction.

- *Do certain women have a greater chance of developing cancer of the breast?*

  1. As women become older the chance increases. More than 80% of women who develop breast cancer are over 40.

  2. If you have a sister or mother with breast cancer, your chances are 2 to 3 times higher of developing cancer. There may be a genetic predisposition.

  3. Women who have had no children, an early onset of menses (before 11), first babies after 30 and late menopause (after 50) are also at greater risk.

  4. There is no evidence that postmenopausal estrogen replacement causes breast cancer.[1]

- *Does estrogen cause cancer of the breast?*

  Estrogen does not seem to be a carcinogen (cancer causer). Dr. R. Don Gambrell, Jr. of the Medical College of Georgia, showed in his studies in 1983 that women on estrogen alone had a lower incidence of breast cancer than women who took no hormones. Women on both estrogen and progestogen had an incidence even lower than that. This same study suggests estrogen and progestogen may even protect against cancer of the breast.

- *What about birth-control pills and cancer of the breast?*

  There is no evidence that birth-control pills increase the risk of breast cancer. They may even decrease the risk.

- *If I develop cancer of the breast, do I have to lose my breast?*

  If you develop cancer of the breast, a lumpectomy (removal of a tumor without other tissue or lymph nodes) may be all that is required. A simple mastectomy (removal of a breast) followed by radiation where indicated gives good results. If your breast must be removed, it's possible that a prosthesis can be inserted in its place with no noticeable loss of contour.

- *My doctor refused to give me estrogen until I had mammography. If estrogen and progesterone do not cause cancer of the breast, why would he insist upon this test?*

  Your doctor is both thorough and cautious. Although there is no proof estrogen causes cancer of the breast, it may increase the

1   Townsend, M. "Management of Breast Cancer." *Clinical Symposia.* 1987. Vol. 39, No. 4: 3-32. (CIBA-Geigy).

spread of cancer when it is present. Your doctor wanted to make certain you did not already have cancer of the breast before prescribing hormones (ERT) for you.

- *You mentioned the increased risk of estrogen-related breast cancer and women who have had it must not take ERT. How would I know if my breast cancer is estrogen-related?*

Although this rule is not absolute, most breast cancers that develop before menopause are estrogen-related. Those breast cancers that develop after menopause, especially 5 years after, are nearly always non-estrogen-dependent.

There are generally two types of breast cancer. The *glandular* rather than the *ductal* is more likely to be estrogen-dependent. Your doctor can tell you which type a cancer is, especially if the tissue was tested for estrogen receptors.

- *Because about two-thirds of breast cancers occur in women over 50, isn't it unnecessary to worry younger women so much about breast cancer?*

Breast cancer is rare under 35, but it does occur. As soon as young women begin intercourse, they are old enough to be taught to check their breasts for cancer. They should also begin to have regular Pap smears and have their first screening mammography at 35.

- *Is there anything I can do to reduce the risk of cancer during menopause and the years to follow?*

1. We have mentioned the importance of regular visits to your doctor. We recommend an annual visit.

2. Report any abnormal bleeding promptly, whether your periods are longer, heavier or irregular. This includes spotting between periods.

3. Decrease your intake of fats, both saturated and unsaturated.

4. Eat high-fiber foods such as fruits, vegetables, whole-grain cereals, corn and rice.

5. Keep your weight normal. Obesity increases your risk of certain kinds of cancer, especially breast and endometrial cancer. Severe underweight can likewise be harmful to your health. Avoid food fads and quackery.

6. Avoid smoking and limit your alcohol intake. These drugs can control your life. Both increase the risk of cancer.

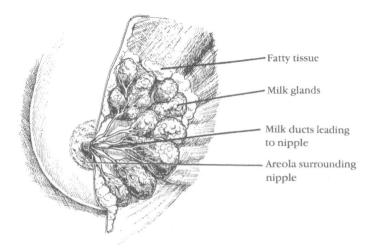

Fatty tissue

Milk glands

Milk ducts leading
to nipple

Areola surrounding
nipple

Structure of a normal breast.

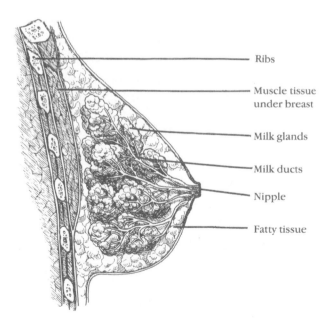

Ribs

Muscle tissue
under breast

Milk glands

Milk ducts

Nipple

Fatty tissue

Side view of normal breast structure.

7. Finally, watch for the warning signs of cancer:

    a. Unexplained weight loss

    b. Unexplained fever, fatigue or pain

    c. Change in bladder or bowel habits

    d. Sores that do not heal

    e. Bleeding or discharge from any source

    f. Thickening or lumps in breasts or anywhere else in body

    g. Indigestion such as heartburn; bloated, queasy stomach; burping; loss of appetite or difficulty swallowing

    h. Change in appearance of any mole or wart

    i. Cough or hoarseness that persists

- *Can you give some other helpful facts about cancer of the breast?*

Here are facts every woman should know about breast cancer:

1. Breast cancer is the second-most-common cancer in women. Since smoking has become so common among women, lung cancer is now more prevalent than breast cancer. Breast cancer will strike one out of every 11 women in their lifetime.

2. About 70 percent of cancers of the breast are first discovered during self-examination. Learn to check yourself for breast cancer. See pages 44–46 for the most effective techniques.

3. Every woman should have a baseline mammogram by 35, repeated at 40, then every 2 years until 50 and every year thereafter. Mammograms detect cancer of the breast long before you can feel it with your fingers. Example: Nancy Reagan was 67 when breast cancer was discovered. If she had failed to have a mammogram, her cancer might have been discovered too late.

4. Cancer of the breast is extremely rare before 30, but becomes more common with age.

5. There is still some dispute among the experts whether women who breast-feed their children may be at slightly less risk for cancer of the breast.

6. If you have breast cancer in your family, especially your mother or sister, you are 2 to 3 times as likely to develop breast cancer. There may be a genetic predisposition. You may need mammograms more often. Check with your doctor.

7. If your menstrual periods began before 12 or if you have a late menopause, you have a greater risk of developing breast cancer.

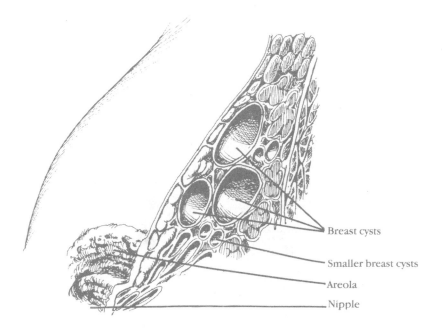

Fibrocystic disease of the breast. There are several cysts and they vary in size. They often enlarge just before a menstrual period and become tender.

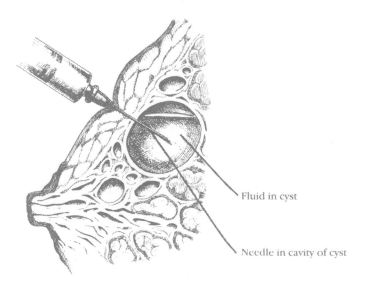

Withdrawal of fluid (or aspiration) from a breast cyst is a simple way to make a diagnosis. If a mass completely disappears after withdrawal of fluid, the problem is solved. If there is still a mass, it must be biopsied.

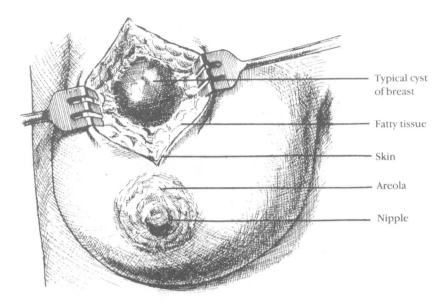

Typical cyst of breast

Fatty tissue

Skin

Areola

Nipple

Typical cyst of the breast is benign. It is often seen in fibrocystic disease of the breast.

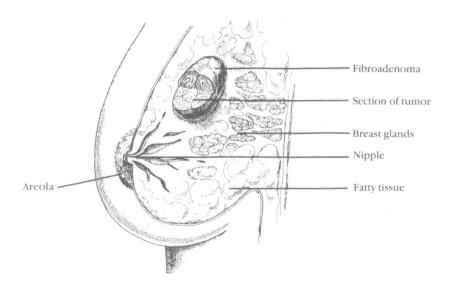

Fibroadenoma

Section of tumor

Breast glands

Nipple

Areola

Fatty tissue

A fibroadenoma is a benign tumor often found in young women between 15 and 30. It is not painful and will not turn into cancer.

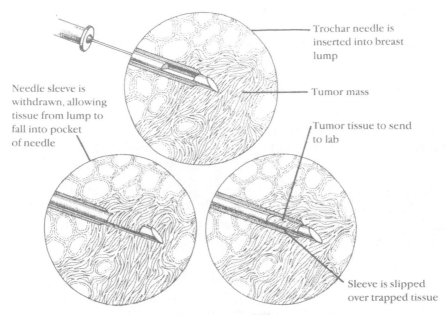

Trochar needle is
inserted into breast
lump

Needle sleeve is
withdrawn, allowing
tissue from lump to
fall into pocket
of needle

Tumor mass

Tumor tissue to send
to lab

Sleeve is slipped
over trapped tissue

*Detailed view of a method of removing breast tissue from a breast
lump by needle biopsy for examination.*

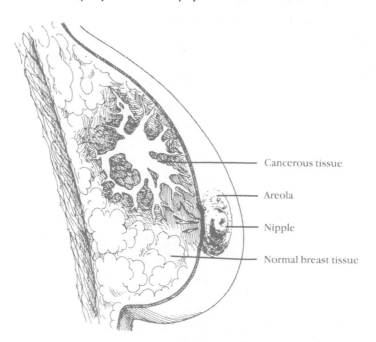

Cancerous tissue

Areola

Nipple

Normal breast tissue

Cancer of the breast beginning to spread.

8. You have a greater risk of breast cancer if you have had no children or if you had your first child late in life. In general, the more children, the lower the risk of breast cancer.

9. Recent information suggests high-fat diets increase the risk of developing breast cancer.

10. Caffeine does not cause cancer of the breast.

11. There is no evidence that postmenopausal estrogen-replacement therapy (ERT) actually causes breast cancer.

- *I had breast cancer at 41. I am now 52 and having severe hot flashes. My doctor mentioned calcitonin injections to relieve these symptoms and to prevent the development of osteoporosis. Will these shots relieve the hot flashes?*

Calcitonin will not relieve hot flashes. It is used to treat osteoporosis. Discuss some alternatives with your doctor—such as Megace® (progestin), clonidine (Catapres®) or possibly Bellergal® to help relieve the hot flashes.

- *Can cancer be cured?*

Yes. Many cancers can be cured by:

  a. Surgery
  b. Radiation therapy
  c. Radioactive substances
  d. Certain drugs

Summary

In conclusion, you may be at greater risk for cancer during and following menopause just because you are older. But you can offset this disadvantage to some extent by being wiser. We have outlined the need for regular, annual visits to your doctor. These visits should include a pelvic examination, a Pap smear (according to schedule) and a breast examination. Breast self-examination is also vital.

Check with your doctor if you have any abnormal uterine bleeding, abnormal vaginal discharge or abdominal or pelvic pain. Remember you pay for the care you receive. But you receive the best care only if you give your doctor a chance to care for you.

If you have multiple sexual contacts, insist your partner use a condom. For additional protection you may want to use one of the vaginal spermicidal creams. This combination may be helpful in protecting against sexually transmitted diseases. The papilloma virus is thought to increase your risk of cervical cancer. The most-recent studies indicate this virus is more serious than herpes as a cause of cervical cancer.

On the positive side, if you follow the simple suggestions we have made, you will find the greatest advance in preventive medicine is your own individual, intelligent vigilance.

4

Vaginal Discharge, Sexually Transmitted Diseases & Menopause

There was a time when *venereal disease* meant either syphilis or gonorrhea. Modern culture and social practices have brought an entirely new set of sex practices and new sexually transmitted diseases.

Chlamydia, unknown until just a few years ago, is now more common than gonorrhea, reaching upwards of 3-million cases each year. Mead & Sweet (1985) say chlamydial infection may be as much as 10 times more common than gonorrhea.

Herpes and AIDS are also newcomers as sexually transmitted diseases. Because of oral and anal sex, additional diseases such as amebiasis and giardiasis have been included as sexually transmitted diseases.

- *Which diseases are considered to be sexually transmitted?*

Because of changes in sexual practices, the list has now been expanded to include the following (according to the American Public Health Association):

AIDS
Amebiasis
Cancer of the cervix
Chancroid
Chlamydial infections
Conjunctivitis due to chlamydia
Cytomegalovirus infections of newborns
Dermatophytosis
Gardnerella vaginalis
Giardiasis
Gonorrhea
Granuloma inguinale

Hepatitis, both A and B
Herpes simplex
Lymphogranuloma venereum
Melioidosis
Mycoplasma hominis
Molluscum contagiosum
Mononucleosis, infectious
Pediculosis
Scabies
Streptoccal infection of the newborn, Group B
Syphilis
T-Mycoplasma (ureaplasma urealyticum)
Trichomoniasis
Venereal warts (condyloma acuminata, papilloma virus)

A rather imposing list!

- *I was so happy to be rid of menstrual periods. But now I have a bothersome discharge my doctor calls* chlamydia. *What is it?*

  Chlamydia is an infection caused by a bacterium called *Chlamydia trachomatis.* Typically, it attacks the urinary tract and genitals of the male and the entire genital tract of the female, except for the vagina. The vagina, for reasons we don't understand, remains immune to the infection. Chlamydia also attacks the urethra (tube from the bladder to the outside) in both sexes.

- *What sort of symptoms does chlamydia cause?*

  Most chlamydial infections cause no symptoms. However, chlamydial infection may cause a stinging and burning sensation in the bladder and urethra, as well as frequent urination. It may cause a heavy mucous-pus discharge from the cervix. If the infection is forced up into the uterus during intercourse, it causes infection of the lining of the uterus (endometritis), which will make your uterus sore to touch.

  From the uterus, the infection progresses outward into the fallopian tubes, where it causes salpingitis (infection of the tubes) and often produces infertility. About 35,000 new cases of infertility each year may be due to chlamydial infection. Chlamydial infection causes more sterility in women than gonorrhea.

- *How does a woman get chlamydial infection?*

  If a man has chlamydial infection in his urethra, his sex partners have at least a 25-percent chance of also developing chlamydial urethritis. Chlamydia is now our most common sexually transmitted disease (formerly known as *venereal disease*).

Chlamydial bacteria attack human cells, enter them and begin to live within the body cells just like a parasite. They are literally swallowed up by the body cells. Yet they continue to grow within the body cell until the cell bursts, releasing additional infectious chlamydial particles that invade other cells and continue the vicious, infectious process.

- *Isn't chlamydial infection just found in younger women?*

No. As long as you are sexually active, you can catch chlamydial infection. It may be more common in younger women who are more active sexually and who may have multiple sex partners.

- *How can I know for sure if I have chlamydial infection?*

A smear, culture and a Microtrak® test are used to make the diagnosis. Several other tests are being studied. If you develop gonorrhea, you should also be tested for chlamydia because chlamydial infection is more common and may coexist with gonorrhea.

- *Is chlamydia considered to be a venereal disease? That seems like such an unpleasant term.*

Yes. These diseases are now called *sexually transmitted diseases*. This means they are *venereal*, as we used to call them.

- *Is there a treatment for chlamydial infection?*

Yes. Most doctors, if they suspect chlamydial infection, will treat you while they are waiting for the test results (assuming they use the culture method of testing). Tetracycline or some other broad-spectrum antibiotic is commonly prescribed and is very effective.

Penicillin is quickly effective in most instances in the treatment of gonorrhea, but it will not cure chlamydial infection. Some doctors prescribe both drugs without waiting for a diagnosis. If you fit into any of the following categories, you should be tested and treated (if positive) for chlamydial infection:

1. If you have a mucopurulent (mucous, containing pus) cervical discharge.

2. If you have *acute urethral syndrome* (frequency, urgency, painful urination and a sterile urine specimen containing pus).

3. If you have a positive test for gonorrhea because chlamydia

so often accompanies gonorrhea.

4. If you have a partner who has either a non-gonorrheal urethritis or a history of a "morning-drip" type of penile discharge.

5. If you have infection of your tubes or ovaries, also called *pelvic inflammatory disease* or *PID*.

- *How long does it take to treat chlamydia?*

  Usually a 10-day treatment with tetracycline will do it. If this fails, you may have to take erythromycin or clindamycin. If that doesn't work, consider the possibility of having been re-infected.

  To be sure you are cured, a culture should be taken after the treatment. It's also important that your partner be treated at the same time, or you will get the disease all over again.

  During treatment, your sex partner should use a condom until a culture proves *both* of you are cured.

- *Are you sure I still have to worry about chlamydial infection even though I am experiencing menopause?*

  Yes. We mentioned anyone who is sexually active may still develop chlamydial infection. But there is another catch: Chlamydial infection may have lain dormant for many years and raise its ugly head at the most inopportune time. In a younger woman this may come when she gives birth to a child. In older women chlamydia may come if the urethra is irritated or if an old pelvic inflammatory disease flares up.

- *Is chlamydia transmitted by kissing?*

  No. Chlamydia is transmitted through mucous membranes such as the eyes (chlamydial eye infection) by sexual contact and to newborns through the birth canal. Chlamydial eye infection is the leading cause of blindness in third-world countries.

  Other contact such as clothing, toilet seats and kissing will not transmit the disease.

- *How long is chlamydia communicable?*

  We don't know. It can lie dormant for years. No one seems to be immune. You can get it again, even if you have had it once and been successfully treated.

- *I am past my menopause and was recently diagnosed as having chlamydial cervicitis. I am widowed and have not been sexually active since my husband's death 2 years ago. How could I have contracted a sexually transmitted disease?*

Recent studies in Japan (T. Nagashima, 1987) and Sweden establish that chlamydia may lie dormant inside cells for a long period of time because a woman's antibodies cannot reach them. Chlamydial organisms could have resided within your cervical cells since the initial infection when your husband was still alive.

Another possibility is primary infection through other mucous membranes, such as your eyes. In such tissues the organisms may also lie dormant for decades. They wait for optimum conditions to enable them to migrate to your cervix where they flare up and cause problems.

- *Is there any way to avoid chlamydia when it is so common?*

First of all, be aware of its presence. Know it is fairly easy and inexpensive to treat. Second, if you have a vaginal discharge or other evidence of infection (pain, fever, etc.) have your doctor check you for this disease. If your sex partner has any penile discharge or evidence of soreness, insist he be checked. Also, insist he wear a condom when you have intercourse.

If you develop chlamydia, inform your sex partners so they can also obtain treatment at the same time.

- *You have said so much about chlamydia and how common it is. Does this mean there is not very much gonorrhea or syphilis anymore?*

Not really. It is just that we know more about chlamydia now than we used to. Many of the so-called *penicillin-resistant* cases of gonorrhea may have been chlamydial infection. If tetracycline had been used to treat these "resistant" cases, many probably would have cleared up immediately.

- *Do you actually see many cases of syphilis anymore?*

Syphilis is primarily a disease of young persons between the ages of 15 and 30. It is more common among the poor and the underprivileged, more in urban than in rural areas and more in males than females.

Since 1957, early venereal syphilis has increased significantly throughout much of the world.

If you develop any of the sexually transmitted diseases or if you have had several sex partners, have a blood test to rule out syphilis and a smear and culture to rule out gonorrhea. Insist your sex partner wash his genitals before and after intercourse. Have him use a condom, just to give you added protection against nearly all of the diseases we have discussed.

As you are aware, syphilis is easily treated with penicillin. It should be diagnosed and treated early, before additional damage is done. The same applies to gonorrhea.

- *Is there a great risk of developing herpes during and after menopause?*

Herpes genitalis knows no age limits. It is the herpes virus type 2 that usually produces genital herpes. It occurs primarily in adults and is sexually transmitted. *HSV 2*, as it is called, is also thought to be a risk factor in cancer of the cervix.

- *How do I know when I have herpes?*

Although the primary reservoir of herpes may be in the cervix, you will feel discomfort on your vulva where small, painful blisters appear. If you have blisters and extremely tender areas on your vulva, suspect herpes 2. Get a checkup by your doctor.

Your doctor will confirm the diagnosis of herpes 2, either by examining scrapings of the lesions under the microscope or by herpes cultures.

- *Is there anything I can do to avoid getting herpes 2 infection? I am divorced, 49-years old but active sexually with several partners.*

1. Limit your intimacy to those sex partners you know very well.

2. Insist your sex partners use a condom.

3. Ask your sex partners if they have herpes.

4. If you develop herpes, tell your sex partners.

5. Never have sex when there is active disease, i.e., when blisters are present.

- *My husband and I occasionally engage in oral sex. He recently developed a cold sore on his lip that has now disappeared. Now I have developed a small blister on my vulva which my doctor states is herpes. Could this possibly have been contracted during our encounter with oral sex?*

Yes. Your own herpes probably came from your husband. Although the virus that causes a cold sore comes from the herpes

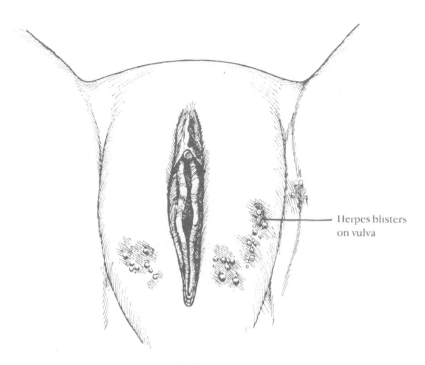

The diagnosis of herpes vaginalis is made with the appearance of cold-sore blisters on the vulva. This disease can be fatal to a newborn.

simplex or herpes-1 virus, it may be transmitted by oral sex or even by hands to the genital area, resulting in blisters in the genital area. Such genital-herpes breakouts are most likely to occur when your resistance is down.

In order to be sure if this is herpes and to determine the type, have your physician determine if this is herpes-1 or herpes-2 virus. This is done by culture and typing.

• *My doctor told me I have herpes blisters on my vulva. My boyfriend denies he has herpes. If this is true, how did I get it?*

Herpes, like many diseases, can be carried by the male partner who may have no symptoms. Just because a male has no *acute outbreak* of a sexually transmitted disease does not mean he is not a carrier of one of these diseases.

Another possibility is you may have contracted the herpes virus months before. It has remained dormant until your immune responses were altered in such a way you now are breaking out. In other words, you may have had a primary herpes infection months ago and did not recognize it. This may be a recurrence of that infection.

Avoid any sexual contact during your active breakout. Have your male partner use a condom for at least 3 weeks *after* your blisters have cleared because they may still be shedding viruses for this long. Acyclovir medications now available in capsules or topical ointment may help force the virus into remission.

Once you have had a known herpes infection, have an annual physical examination with a Pap smear to detect any early changes that suggest cancer of either your cervix or your vulva.

- *Is there any cure for herpes 2?*

Not at the present time. There are some medications that help relieve the discomfort and promote healing of the blisters. Some preparations are thought to help in quieting down the disease. Discuss this with your doctor. Acyclovir seems to reduce the incidence of recurrence or flare-ups.

Herpes may flare up only once a year in some women, every month or two in others. Acute herpes late in a mother's pregnancy can cause a fatal infection in her newborn delivered through the birth canal.

When you have blisters, you should stay away from newborns, children with eczema or burns and those individuals who must take immunosuppressant drugs. Immunosuppressant drugs are taken by people who may have had organ transplants.

- *I recently married (at 46). I have developed lesions on my vulva and around the anal area. My doctor tells me these are venereal warts. How did I get these? What can I do to get rid of them? Are they likely to recur?*

Condylomata acuminata (venereal warts) are caused by a virus of the papilloma family. It is a sexually transmitted disease. You probably caught it from your new husband. Although he shows no visible signs of the disease, he could still be a carrier. Frequently the lesions are high in the urethra or even in the bladder. But they still serve as the source of the infection. He should be examined and treated by a urologist.

Most of these lesions respond well to a medication containing podophyllin.

If they are extremely large, they can also be removed with cryosurgery (frozen) or removed by laser beams. In most instances they do not recur if they have been adequately treated. If your immune response has been altered by pregnancy or some illness, the warts might recur.

Certain strains of papilloma virus increase your risk for developing vulvar and cervical cancer. If you have had condylomata, get a checkup at least once a year and have a Pap smear because of the increased risk of developing cancer of the cervix.

Any abnormal-appearing sore or lesion on your vulva should be checked by your doctor and biopsied, if necessary, to rule out cancer, especially at menopause and thereafter.

- *What about trichomonas infection? Is this considered to be sexually transmitted? I have always understood it is very common.*

Trichomonas infection is extremely common. It is definitely a sexually transmitted disease. Typically it is ping-ponged back and forth between sexual partners, even between a husband and wife who are strictly faithful to each other.

Trichomonas infection may not show any symptoms, or it can cause severe itching and profuse discharge. Found mostly in adults in the 16- to 35-year-old group, it may also occur in menopausal women.

Trichomonas infection is due to a protozoan with a tail that propels it rapidly. This infection causes a very-profuse, foul-smelling, foamy, yellowish discharge.

If you develop trichomonas infection, both you and your sex partner should take treatment at the same time. Otherwise you will recontaminate and infect each other over and over again. The best and only drug that is effective is metronidazole. Flagyl® is one of the well-known brand names. It should be taken simultaneously by you and your partner.

If one round of treatment does not clear up the infection, both you and your sex partner must repeat the treatment all over again. Treatment lasts only a week. You'll find it beneficial to abstain from intercourse during this time.

- *After taking penicillin for a sore throat last week, I developed a terrible itching and a whitish, curd-like discharge. What could this be?*

When you take penicillin or other types of antibiotics for an infection, it also removes the normal bacteria from your vagina, allowing yeast to flourish. The symptoms you describe are typical of a yeast infection. It would be wise for you to have your doctor confirm this diagnosis and prescribe treatment for you.

In the future when you take penicillin or any other antibiotic, remind your doctor you developed a yeast infection the last time you took an antibiotic. He will undoubtedly prescribe antifungal vaginal medication which will prevent your developing yeast infection next time. Once you have developed yeast infection, a short course of antifungal vaginal medication will promptly clear up the yeast and relieve your symptoms.

Women with diabetes are also prone to develop yeast infection. If you have diabetes, be aware that the thick, curd-like discharge so typical of yeast infection can be successfully treated.

- *My problem is not too much discharge or any irritation from a discharge. My problem seems to be I have NO discharge! Intercourse is very painful because I am so dry. My husband thinks it is because I am not aroused, but this is not so. What can we do about this?*

As you near your menopause, less estrogen is secreted. Therefore there is less secretion with arousal. In fact, there will be less discharge all the time. For intercourse the best thing you can do is use an artificial, water-soluble lubricant such as Replens®, H-R®, K-Y® or Lubafax® lubricating jelly. Or. you could use vaginal suppositories such as Lubrin® Vaginal Lubricating Inserts.

Estrogen vaginal cream is prescribed for many women after menopause because it stimulates the mucous membranes of the vagina to thicken. As these membranes thicken, they are less subject to irritation and chafing, especially with intercourse. However, estrogen cream is a poor lubricant for intercourse.

- *What is AIDS?*

AIDS stands for *Acquired Immune Deficiency Syndrome,* a condition in which a blood-borne virus attacks and destroys the body's immune system.

- *How is AIDS transmitted?*

AIDS is most likely to pass from one person to another during anal intercourse. It can also be transmitted by vaginal intercourse, by contaminated hypodermic needles and syringes, and by contaminated blood transfusions. It can also pass from an infected mother to her child, either while she is carrying it or during delivery.

- *What about oral sex transmitting AIDS?*

It may be possible, but so far there is no definitive evidence.

- *Isn't AIDS a disease of male homosexuals?*

No. Although this is the group most at risk, bisexuals, prostitutes, intravenous drug users, hemophiliacs who had many transfusions before adequate testing of blood was available and now spouses of all these groups are at increased risk.

In Haiti and Africa, AIDS has become a heterosexual disease. A similar trend is developing all over the world, including in the United States and Canada.

- *What actually causes AIDS?*

AIDS is caused by a blood-borne virus that attacks and eventually destroys the body's immune system. These viruses take over certain cells in the body and interrupt their genetic functioning. AIDS victims die of some "opportunistic" infection such as pneumonia that takes advantage of the body's inability to defend itself from infection.

- *Is AIDS always fatal?*

This appears to be the case. At present there is no cure and no vaccine, but research is progressing rapidly. Now that we know its cause, we feel certain either preventive vaccines or actual cures will eventually be discovered.

- *Is AIDS easy to catch?*

No. The virus is not transmitted by air or water as most diseases are. Nor does it seem to be transmitted by casual contact or via inanimate objects.

It is transmitted by intimate sexual contact, by contaminated needles, from mother to baby or through blood transfusions from infected individuals. Most children diagnosed as having AIDS are born to AIDS-infected parents. The rest have hemophilia and have received many transfusions before adequate testing of blood for AIDS was developed.

Only about 7 percent of AIDS cases have been traced to heterosexual transmission, but this percentage is increasing. It appears easier to transmit from man to woman than from woman to man. Prostitutes are more likely to be infected because of multiple sex partners. They are also more likely to be using intravenous drugs.

- *Can AIDS be transmitted by casual contact such as a handshake, cough or touching a toilet?*

  No. AIDS is hard to contract. No one should be isolated because he or she has AIDS. Children should not be barred from school because they have AIDS. AIDS virus has been found in saliva, but not in sufficient quantity to cause infection, even if a child should be bitten by another child with AIDS.

- *Can I get AIDS from mosquito or bedbug bites?*

  No case of AIDS has ever been traced to insect bites. If this were the case, AIDS would quickly spread all over the world.

- *I am going to have a hysterectomy soon and am concerned about having a transfusion because of the risk of AIDS. How safe is blood in the blood bank?*

  We now have excellent methods for screening the blood in blood banks. A recent trend has been to take some of your own blood a few weeks before surgery and keep it in readiness in case you require a transfusion. This eliminates the threat of diseases being conveyed by transfusion. Your risk of contracting AIDS by transfusion is less than 1 in 100,000.

- *Can I get AIDS from donating blood?*

  No. All equipment is carefully sterilized so you cannot contract any infection from donating blood.

- *If my husband tests positive for AIDS, does that mean he has the disease?*

  No. But it does mean he has been exposed to it and has developed antibodies to it. At the present time no one knows what percentage of antibody-positive people will go on to develop full-blown AIDS. It may be years before we know the answer to this question.

&.   &.   &.

Unless a cure is found, AIDS is thought by most of the medical community to be the most serious public-health problem facing the Western world today.

In the meantime, you should also be tested. Insist your husband use a condom when you have intercourse.

- *How common is AIDS among women?*

Of the 25,650 AIDS cases confirmed in the United States by the Centers for Disease Control as of October 1986, 1,708 or nearly 7 percent were women. More than half of these women are intravenous drug users, 9.5 percent contracted the disease after blood transfusions. About 27 percent seem to have been infected by heterosexual contact.

Of 300,000 young military recruits screened by Walter Reed Army Institute of Research, 1.5 per 1,000 showed signs of infection by the virus causing AIDS. The ratio between men and women was 2.5 for men to 1 for women. Women are increasingly at risk for AIDS.

Admittedly these are younger women. This may be due to greater sexual activity and more promiscuity among the young. Any woman who has multiple sexual contacts risks developing AIDS.

- *I have heard AIDS is a disease of the young. Do I still have to worry about contracting this disease if I am of menopausal age?*

No one, regardless of age, is immune to the disease. If you have several sex partners and any of them is bisexual or a drug user, you are at increased risk for developing AIDS.

- *An article in the newspaper said AIDS is now showing up in heterosexual couples. Is this true?*

Unless you are using drugs through intravenous injections, your risk is nil for developing AIDS. This assumes you and your sex partner are faithful to each other. The only exception would be if one of you had contracted AIDS a long time ago.

- *Can AIDS be passed from woman to woman?*

In women whose relationship is sexual, it may be possible just as it is possible between a man and a woman. There has been no reported case in which this has happened.

- *My husband has occasional affairs. I have tolerated these because I love him so much. Do I have to worry about the possibility of his catching AIDS and giving it to me?*

Yes, you certainly do. It may pay you to have periodic screening tests for AIDS. Insist he have these same tests. He may catch the disease and pass it on to you. Insist he use a condom.

Remember AIDS is not the only sexually transmitted disease. Your husband could bring home an entire bag of diseases. Look again at the list on pages 57 and 58. Herpes, for instance, has no cure. Some of these diseases, such as the papilloma virus, known as *condyloma acuminata*, increase your chances of developing cancer of the cervix and even cancer of the vulva later in life.

A monogamous relationship is the safest one as far as sexually transmitted diseases are concerned.

- *Will condoms protect me from getting AIDS?*

Condoms help, but the best protection is to maintain a monogamous relationship with someone who does not have AIDS.

- *Articles continue to appear in the newspapers about new discoveries and new research on AIDS. Some of them sound optimistic about these new drugs. Is AIDS still incurable?*

As of this time (1991), AIDS is still incurable and must be considered fatal.

There are perhaps 2-million people in the United States who show a positive test for AIDS but have no clinical symptoms of the disease *yet*. Their future is uncertain because they could develop the disease any time in the years to come.

5

Sex in Menopause

Estrogen decline begins months prior to the menopause and may result in changes in sexual function for many women. These changes become more pronounced as the estrogen deficiency progresses. Estrogen level has a direct impact on sexual arousal, sexual desire and frequency of intercourse. Estrogen-sensitive cells are located throughout the nervous and cardiovascular systems. Loss of estrogen results in decreased blood flow and nerve response during sexual activity.

The common sexual complaints of menopausal women are dyspareunia (dry, painful vagina with intercourse), decreased clitoral sensitivity, decrease in orgasmic frequency, decrease in orgasm intensity, decrease in sexual desire and decrease in frequency of intercourse (once a month or less).

The physiologic changes that cause problems with sexual function for the woman can significantly affect her male partner's ability to get and maintain an erection.

Sexual function will improve or return to the premenopausal status of functioning when women are put on estrogen-replacement therapy (ERT). If sex was satisfying before menopause, it should continue to be satisfying after menopause.[1]

- *Intercourse makes my vagina crack and bleed so I avoid it. This causes a strain on my marriage. What can I do?*

  As estrogen levels fall during menopause it is normal for mucous membranes of the vagina and the skin around the vulva to become thinner, dryer and more sensitive to irritation. As a result of this dryness, the tissues may crack and bleed, especially with intercourse. Pain with intercourse is called *dyspareunia*.

  Although most of this irritation is due to loss of estrogen,

1 Sorrel, D.M. "Sexuality and Menopause." *Obstetrics and Gynecology.* 1990. 75:26S.

infection must be considered. Your doctor can test for yeast, trichomonas, chylamydia, beta streptococcus and other suspected infections and treat accordingly.

Vaginal lubricants—Replens®, K-Y®, H-R®—will provide some immediate relief from dyspareunia. Estrogen vaginal creams and/or estrogen by mouth or patch over several months will restore the vaginal and vulval tissue integrity.

- *Is it true an active sex life will slow down the changes in the vagina which occur due to decreasing estrogen?*

Yes. If intercourse is discontinued, the tissues have a greater tendency to shrink, thus shortening and narrowing the vagina. If a woman has not had sex for several years and then resumes sex postmenopausally, she will most certainly require ERT (estrogen-replacement therapy). The therapy may include estrogen vaginal cream. It may take several months and possibly up to two years to get the vaginal tissues back to sufficient resiliency to overcome discomfort during sex.

- *I have just resumed sex after several years of living alone. If my vagina has now progressed to actual scarring or shrinking causing severe pain with intercourse, can I expect these tissues to return to normal by using estrogen?*

To normal, no. Scarring and shrinking will not disappear. Normal folds of the vagina will not return. You may and should expect resiliency to return to the point you can have normal, enjoyable sex without discomfort, but it will take time.

- *What about using estrogen vaginal cream as a lubricant for intercourse?*

Estrogen vaginal cream is unsatisfactory as a lubricant for intercourse. First of all, estrogen vaginal cream will not be pleasant or even acceptable by your sex partner as a vaginal lubricant because it is messy. Secondly, although estrogen vaginal cream is a form of ERT, its dosage is uncertain. It will not provide sufficient estrogen for complete estrogen replacement therapy. Thirdly, it may take many months of estrogen vaginal cream alone to solve your dyspareunia (painful intercourse) completely. Usually, additional estrogen is necessary to reverse the atrophic changes in your vaginal mucous membranes. Read about lubricating jellies and vaginal suppositories, page 81.

- *I stopped menstruating last year at 49. It seems to take me longer to reach a climax now than it used to. Is this normal?*

  With menopause it is common to find sexual arousal and orgasm come a little slower, but satisfaction will continue if you are willing to put forth the effort. You may also find your husband is having the same response. Estrogen therapy should result in improvement or even a return of your function to the premenopausal state.

  Masters and Johnson (1966), the sex therapists, claim about 50 percent of couples either now have or will have sexual problems. But that does not mean they cannot solve them if they are willing to be patient with each other and try to work through these problems. If you can't talk them out, get some help from your physician. If this fails, you may need to see a sex counselor.

- *Is it normal to expect a certain loss of libido after menopause?*

  Yes, due to the estrogen deficiency, but everyone has a different experience in this regard. Many women experience a lessened libido or one that responds more slowly to arousal. These same women often find they experience as much or more joy with sex if their partners will be patient with them.

  Often the nature and meaning of sex and intimacy change as women enter midlife. They may find more joy in embracing, kissing, cuddling and certain types of fondling. In general, women retain their libido better than men after midlife. It is not uncommon for some women to experience increased libido after the threat of pregnancy or the need for contraception is over.

  When pressures of time and family are no longer present, there is time for relaxation during sex and prolonged stimulation becomes less of a problem. Don't make the mistake of thinking sex is only for the young!

- *Does estrogen sometimes restore lost libido?*

  Yes. There should be an improvement or a return to the premenopausal status. But you should also discuss the sexual relationship with your partner. Discuss the problem with your doctor. If you still have a problem after six months on estrogen-replacement therapy, then try small doses of testosterone. If both of these fail, you may need consultation with a sex counselor.

- *I am 55 and so far have not taken estrogen. I have reached the point I feel I am well past menopause. I have a little dryness and tenderness in my vagina, but I can handle this with a lubricating jelly. Is it certain these conditions will become worse as I get older if I don't take estrogen?*

Dr. Lila Nachtigall (1986) is one of the most reliable authorities on menopausal changes. She says you will almost certainly have uncomfortable intercourse if you do not take estrogen post-menopausally. This stems from increasing dryness and thinning of the vaginal mucous membranes.

It may take 5, 10 or even 15 years for these changes to occur, but they are going to happen.

- *Since going through menopause 3 years ago, I have noticed an increase in my desire for sex. I admit part of this desire is due to the freedom from worry of pregnancy. My dilemma is my husband has difficulty obtaining and maintaining an erection. Any suggestions?*

This is a time when you need to be patient with your husband. A man's sexual desire and ability to reach orgasm peak at about age 18 to 20. Some men notice a tapering off during their 30s and a marked decrease during their 40s.

Because men tend to equate their sexual ability with masculinity, any decrease in this regard threatens their self-esteem and confidence. If not handled carefully and understandingly, this can become a psychologically vicious circle. The more he worries, the more difficulty a man has. The more difficulty he has with sex, the more he worries.

A sympathetic and understanding wife can make the difference between success and failure in many cases. First of all, learn to talk together. Take time for each other.

Your children are probably gone. Your schedules may not be as hectic as they used to be. Don't try as hard and don't hurry. Take time to be affectionate. Let intercourse come as a natural part of that affection on its own, rather than a goal that must be reached.

- *Just a year ago, at age 44, I had my fallopian tubes tied. Since then I have not been able to have an orgasm. My husband and I are frustrated because we love each other very much. Is this common?*

This is fairly common. It also happens occasionally when a man has a vasectomy. Sometimes when a woman has a tubal ligation, her husband becomes impotent. This phenomenon is psychological and may be due to the incorrect idea such an operation renders a woman less feminine or a man less masculine. Both ideas are medically and physiologically unfounded, but your mind thinks otherwise.

It is common for this to occur if you have a hysterectomy. Yet many women notice a great increase in their sex drive and sexual response after a hysterectomy or a tubal ligation. They no longer have to concern themselves with pregnancy.

Perhaps understanding will help. Possibly taking more time for stimulation will produce the desired result. Most cases like yours we have seen have been temporary and have responded to patience and understanding on the part of both partners. If your problem continues, seek sexual counseling.

- *I am embarrassed to admit it, but I have never had an orgasm in 25 years of marriage. I have faked it and I doubt my husband knows it. Is it too late for me to learn?*

It is never too late to learn. One of our patients left our office angry—at herself. After achieving success, she felt upset with herself because she had, as she said, "wasted" over 20 years of marriage, during which time she could have enjoyed sex.

Both you and your husband should seek sex counseling. With your good attitude, you will undoubtedly become orgasmic.

- *When we were younger I was able to climax easily during intercourse without any other stimulation. I am now 48 and notice I require more stimulation of the clitoris to achieve orgasm. Is that normal and will it continue to become more difficult to climax?*

Many women find their sexual response lessens as their estrogen levels decline. Because estrogen has a direct impact on sexual arousal and ability to climax, see your doctor to be sure your estrogen levels are adequate. A blood estradiol level can help determine whether you are getting enough estrogen. You are to be complimented that both of you resorted to stimulation of the clitoris to help your response.

Take time to discuss your relationship and inform your husband as to your response. You can help each other if you are able to

٭ ٭ ٭

In general, you should expect your relationship with your partner to remain the same as before menopause. If sex has been satisfying in the past, it should continue to be satisfying in the future.

coach one another in your intercourse.

Changes in sexual reactions and response become problems only when they are not talked about.

- *Since my menopause 5 years ago I've noticed I am not completely relaxed after one climax. If my husband helps me reach an additional climax, I am able to relax and sleep better. My husband seems to be having just the opposite response. What shall we do?*

It sounds as though you are already taking care of the situation when you say your husband helps you reach your second orgasm.

There is no harm in reaching multiple orgasms. This is extremely common in women, especially younger women. Your husband should feel no obligation to have ejaculations to keep up with your orgasms. He probably doesn't and couldn't. Obviously you have worked out your problem. You need only to be told you have a healthy sexual relationship.

- *Is there really such a thing as the G spot in women that is super-sensitive?*

In about 1950 Dr. Ernest Grafenberg, a gynecologist, described a small area in the upper vagina directly beneath the pubic bone that, when stimulated, produced intense sexual response. Some physicians have agreed and supposedly reproduced these results. Others doubt the existence of such an area.

We suggest you and your husband or sex partner explore this upper, outer portion of your vagina with the hope you discover something that will heighten your response during intercourse.

- *Since age 20 I have been a heavy smoker (3 packs per day). Now that I am in my late 40s I am noticing a definite slowing of sexual response. I worry about menopause making this response even slower. Does smoking really have any effect upon sexual response?*

Smokers have lower levels of estrogen which can certainly have an impact on sexual response. Also, smokers experience menopause 1 to 2 years earlier than non-smokers.[2]

Because smoking has so many other negative effects, why don't you quit with the hope your sexual response will improve? There are many stop-smoking clinics to help you.

2   Gold, E.B. "Smoking and the Menopause." *Menopause Management.* Nov. 1990. Vol. 3, No. 3:9-11.

- *Now I am in my 50s, I look back and see I have always had a problem becoming aroused. I do not drink but I am wondering if a few drinks would relax me and help me to become aroused more easily?*

It is true a few drinks may help you relax. Whether or not these drinks would help you become aroused is questionable. Some people find they cannot respond sexually if they have a few drinks. There is also the problem that a few drinks make some people drunk.

There's no way to determine ahead of time who might become addicted to alcohol, so you may find it better to leave well enough alone. Instead, try a little exploring with your sex partner to discover just what does arouse you best and easiest. Quicker is not always better. Maybe you require more time. Alcohol is not a stimulant—it's a depressant that could slow you down even more.

- *Some magazine articles and also some newer books are referring to supersex to describe the changes ERT will make in a postmenopausal woman. Is this an exaggeration?*

Without estrogen nearly every woman will experience changes in her entire body and especially in her vagina. A woman without estrogen may experience loss of desire and diminished sexual responsiveness and her vaginal tissues will undergo thinning and drying. As this process continues, the vagina may shrink, shorten and become less resilient. When these changes are combined with lack of lubrication, uncomfortable sex will probably result.

It is true these changes can be stopped and even reversed by estrogen in any form. As vaginal cream, estrogen has a direct effect on the vaginal tissues. The effective dose is more difficult to ascertain than when given orally or as a skin patch. Most doctors prescribe a combination of these methods.

Estrogen will provide improvement or even a return to the premenopausal levels of desire and responsiveness. But it will not produce what was not there before menopause. In other words, don't expect your libido to be greater than it was before menopause. Estrogen may restore what may have been temporarily lost by the discomfort of thinning and drying of these tissues.

These changes are slow to occur when estrogen is lost. It may likewise take some time to obtain complete relief when estrogen is provided by ERT. Allow several weeks or even up to two years for your vaginal tissues to return to normal. Unlike the changes of osteoporosis, vaginal-tissue changes can be reversed and eventually returned almost to normal.

- *Aren't there some aphrodisiacs that will stimulate both my husband and me now we are getting older and slowing down?*

There are many aphrodisiacs (sex stimulators). The most famous is Spanish Fly. Spanish Fly is not a medicine. It is an irritant that supposedly causes sexual stimulation because it causes inflammation in your genitals and bladder.

Like other aphrodisiacs, Spanish Fly is toxic and can produce damage to your organs and even death. The best aphrodisiac of all is caring. At your age you have more time than ever. Talk to each other as you express unhurried love. Even though your responses may have slowed, they can be more meaningful and satisfying.

- *My nipples have always been inverted— even more so now I am experiencing menopause. I find this embarrassing when I make love. Can anything be done about this?*

We can tell you is it is so common it is normal. Also, you will notice as your nipples are stimulated, they become erect and are no longer inverted. When women are nursing, they first stimulate their inverted nipples to make them erect for the baby to take hold.

You may find you can stimulate the nipples by massaging them and cause them to become erect before you begin to make love. Inverted nipples should be no cause for embarrassment.

- *Since my hysterectomy I have had almost no desire for sex. Is this my unhappy lot for the rest of my life?*

First of all, you should understand a hysterectomy (removal of uterus and cervix) does not remove any of the organs that affect or lessen your desire for sex or your ability to climax. This response is definitely an emotional one. It is something you can correct. Some men are temporarily impotent following a vasectomy, possibly because they can no longer father a child.

Take plenty of time with your husband to kiss and caress. Forget about desire or ability to climax. Simply love and explore. The lack of response is temporary and will change in time. Only rarely is it necessary to administer small amounts of testosterone to restore sexual desire.

• *At 45 I am going to have a hysterectomy because of heavy bleeding. My doctor has not been able to control the bleeding with a D&C or medicine. My doctor has left it up to me about removing my ovaries. Do you think this will affect my sex life?*

Removal of your ovaries should not affect your sex life if you are placed on adequate estrogen following surgery. If your sexual response was okay before surgery, it will be okay afterward and vice versa. You have 4 or 5 years left in which your ovaries should continue to function and secrete estrogen. If you have your ovaries removed, you will immediately undergo surgical menopause. You will begin to have menopausal symptoms (hot flashes, insomnia, nervousness, etc.) unless you are placed on ERT.

On the other hand, if your ovaries are left intact, you are faced with the slight possibility of cancer in them. Although cancer of the ovaries is not common, it does occur. It is appropriately called the *silent cancer,* because it rarely causes any symptoms until it has progressed so far it may be difficult to treat. Perhaps because ovarian cancer is silent, it is second only to cancer of the breast as a cause of cancer death in women. In the United States over 20,000 die each year of ovarian cancer.

Add this to the fact you can and probably will take estrogen replacement after menopause anyway. This will not only relieve menopausal symptoms, but will also prevent osteoporosis (loss of calcium from the bone) and cardiovascular disease. You must debate whether it would indeed be better to have your ovaries removed at age 45 and be rid of the risk of cancer in them. See page 41.

It is normal for your doctor to leave this decision up to you. Every woman has her own special feelings about her ovaries and about taking hormones. As physicians, we lean toward "prophylactic" removal of the ovaries whenever hysterectomy is done after 45.

• *I have had 5 children. I must admit my vagina feels somewhat loose during intercourse. Can anything be done about this?*

Yes, Dr. Arnold Kegel developed some exercises to strengthen the muscles that support the vagina, bladder and rectum. These consist of two exercises:

1. Tighten or squeeze your vagina and your rectum by drawing these muscles up into the vagina. Squeeze your buttocks together and hold in this position for 5 to 10 seconds. Then relax and repeat the exercise as many times as you can, gradually working up to 100 or more times each day.

This exercise can be performed while sitting, standing, stooping or whatever. You can do it at work, at home and while you are doing other things. It may take hundreds of repetitions. You will eventually notice a definite tightening ability in these tissues. As these vaginal muscles are strengthened, your intercourse will improve.

2. When passing urine, practice starting and stopping the stream as many times as you can. This exercise will strengthen the muscles around your urethra and give you better control over your bladder. Women who lose their urine when coughing, sneezing, straining or even laughing will notice a definite improvement in control of their urine. But it may require several months of conscientious exercise.

If you still lose your urine on straining, keep in mind a bladder-urethra repair and rectocele (hernia of rectum into vagina) repair can and should be done. It can be carried out at the same time you are having a hysterectomy. These are very successful operations. Actually both cystocele (hernia of bladder through vagina) and rectocele are repaired at the same time. Rectocele repair also tightens the vagina for intercourse. See pages 185–189.

- *You mentioned testosterone would stimulate sexual desire. Couldn't I take this all the time?*

Testosterone is the male sex hormone. If taken in large amounts, it will cause growth of unwanted facial hair and a lowering of your voice. If you don't mind these and a few other unpleasant side effects, you can take it.

Tiny amounts of testosterone will, however, help stimulate sexual desire in certain women. It should not and does not have to be continued indefinitely.

- *I am not married but I have been very active sexually. At 52 I am scheduled to have a hysterectomy. Will a sex partner be able to tell I have had my uterus removed?*

If you have an abdominal hysterectomy, there will be an abdominal scar. This scar could indicate any one of several operations. A vaginal hysterectomy also leaves a scar, but it is concealed within the vagina. Unless your partner explores the vagina to feel the cervix, he will not know you have had a hysterectomy unless you tell him.

- *I am 48 and beginning to notice a few hot flashes, although my menstrual periods continue to be regular. My problem is there seems to be less lubrication in my vagina. In fact, it is often too dry for satisfactory intercourse. What do you suggest?*

This is both common and normal at this time in life. There are two ways you might handle the situation. First of all, you could use a good lubricant.

In general, petroleum jelly is unsatisfactory. It seems not only messy, but it may decrease sensation. Replens®, H-R®, K-Y® or Lubafax® lubricating jelly can be used in small amounts and is acceptable to most couples. Or, you could use vaginal suppositories such as Lubrin® Vaginal Lubricating Inserts.

Another approach is to use a small amount of estrogen vaginal cream 2 to 3 times a week. Over time this will stimulate your own natural vaginal secretions. The problem is that estrogen has other effects and could alter your menstrual periods. It should not be used unless prescribed and supervised by your doctor. You will probably require more estrogen by mouth or by skin patch to cause the necessary changes in your vagina.

As you get older, your genital tissues will not only be drier but also thinner and more subject to irritation. Lubrication is important to avoid discomfort and also injury during intercourse.

Be sure vaginal infections and allergens are not a factor.

- *Since my vaginal hysterectomy and bladder repair 4 years ago I have been in excellent health, especially as far as bladder control and rectal support are concerned. I recently remarried. My vagina is too small for comfortable intercourse—almost too painful for orgasm. Is this likely to get worse? If it does, it will ruin my marriage.*

Following your surgery, healing took place by scar formation. This is nature's way of healing. However, with scarring, there is also narrowing. This is what has taken place in your vagina.

If you persist with intercourse, you may expect your vagina to stretch and eventually accommodate the movements of intercourse very well. For now, employ water-soluble vaginal-lubricants freely, see page 81. Also ask your doctor about estrogen vaginal creams, which will further soften and thicken the membranes lining your vagina. You may also need to work with vaginal dilators for a few weeks. Your doctor will instruct you on their use.

If pain during intercourse is too severe, you could use an anesthetic jelly such as Lidocaine® a half hour before intercourse. You should remove all of the ointment before making love so that it will not produce numbness in your husband's penis.

- *Since menopause I have noticed it takes more stimulation to arouse me. My husband has suggested I buy a vibrator to help. Are these instruments effective and are they harmful?*

First of all, it is normal to find you take longer to become aroused. You have probably noticed the same thing about your husband.

A vibrator may be helpful, and it will not harm you. Many couples find a vibrator hastens initial arousal so they can proceed with coitus without further need of help. Still others find it will help a woman who did not climax during intercourse to achieve her climax afterward.

Experimentation will quickly demonstrate what helps you most.

- *My husband had a heart-bypass operation, but the doctor now tells him he is OK. In fact, he is exercising rather vigorously now. I still have a fear he might have another heart attack—especially when we are making love. How dangerous is it to have intercourse after a heart attack?*

If your doctor has given him the go-ahead for exercise and especially vigorous exercise, you do not have to worry. You will probably find the relaxation and relief from stress that orgasm affords will more than compensate for any physical strain during intercourse.

- *Does exercise help or hinder the sexual response I could achieve during love making? I seem to be tired most of the time.*

Fatigue will cool sexual response and desire quicker than almost anything. Rest is essential, but good physical condition may be just as important.

Too many people of both sexes give up exercise as they get older. They gain weight and become sedentary. One of the best ways to improve sexual desire and response is to improve your general physical condition.

If you have not been active and exercising, do not begin right away with intense reconditioning. Begin with short walks, taking particular note of any shortness of breath, easy fatigue or chest pain. If you have not had a physical examination recently, check with your doctor to see how much exercise you should undertake.

We can assure you as your endurance and general condition improve so will your sexual desire and ability.

- *My husband has always had trouble waiting for me to climax. It spoils it for me when he leaves me unfulfilled. I know it is something that probably should have been corrected early in our married life, but I still would like help at this (menopausal) age.*

It is never too late to improve. Ingrained habits may be more difficult to break, but that does not mean improvement is impossible. What you have described is called *premature ejaculation,* a so-called *conditioned reflex* that may or may not have begun with rushed, stressed intercourse.

Premature ejaculation is sometimes an emotional response that becomes worse the harder you try to overcome it. For instance, merely while trying to arouse his wife, a man may ejaculate, then feel terrible about "letting his wife down." The next time he is even more stressed because he is worrying about having "failed" the last time.

Even though neither partner desires it this way, it may help for you to stimulate yourself prior to intercourse. This will speed up your response when you do have intercourse. Once you help your husband overcome his problem, this may no longer be necessary.

Next, both of you should realize it is not necessary and, in fact, may be uncommon for couples to climax simultaneously. This idea of mutual, simultaneous orgasm may be portrayed in books and movies as the expected result. In actuality it is simply not so.

Some men help their partners climax first simply by stimulation, then penetrate and have ejaculation with or without a second climax by the woman. Other couples find it works better the other way around. Simply remember every couple is different. What seems normal and satisfying for you may not be for someone else.

Some women prefer not to climax every time they make love. They love to be held, to be caressed, to be cared for and cared about, but they do not feel like climaxing every time. Nor should either partner feel stressed if this occurs. If men insist upon a climax by their partner every time, they may be asking for resistance and perhaps loss of desire by their mate.

Especially if a man's urge is considerably greater than that of his wife, she may elect to meet his needs and enjoy doing so if she is not required to climax when she does not want to.

Masters and Johnson (1966), recognized authorities on sexual problems, have developed a technique for premature ejaculation that has proved to be extremely successful. But it requires close communication between you and your husband.

With you facing your husband, the foreplay continues as usual with attention focused on stimulating you almost to the point of orgasm with one exception. If your husband feels he is about to ejaculate prematurely or at least before you are ready, he lets you know.

You then employ what Masters and Johnson call the *squeeze technique*. Grasp the penis between your thumb and the first two fingers of your same hand. Place your thumb on the underside of his penis, just where the shaft ends and the head of the penis begins. Place your two fingers on the opposite side of the penis with one finger on each side of the ridge that separates the shaft from the head of the penis.

By squeezing the penis rather firmly for 3 or 4 seconds, your husband will lose his urge to ejaculate momentarily and may lose part of his erection. However, you can promptly manipulate him back to full erection again. If he again feels he must ejaculate before you are ready, you may repeat the procedure.

Even if your husband has already penetrated and feels he cannot resist ejaculation, you may have to have him withdraw and employ the squeeze technique.

Usually premature ejaculation is more common earlier in marriage with the husband gaining better control as he gets older.

The only problem with using the squeeze technique at your age might come if your husband is having difficulty obtaining and maintaining an erection. Communication will dictate whether the technique is necessary or appropriate in your particular case. In many instances, this maneuver has helped re-establish confidence in both partners as they overcome premature ejaculation.

- *I have always required clitoral stimulation to achieve orgasm. Recently I have read vaginal orgasm is preferred to clitoral orgasm. Is this true?*

According to Masters and Johnson (1966), either is satisfactory. Indications are that there is no difference. You are wise to do what seems best for you and your partner regardless of what the so-called *sex manuals* say.

We do feel it wise for you to be informed about your own anatomy and how your organs function. You may find it will help to use a mirror to inspect and learn about yourself.

- *I have had a mastectomy and feel very sensitive about my appearance. In fact, I have a problem even permitting my husband to look at my chest.*

First of all, if you have a caring husband, he loves you with or without your breasts. He will be the best one to assure you of this, and he has probably already done so.

If your own self-esteem seems threatened, talk to your doctor about the possibility of plastic surgery to insert an implant. These devices are soft and feel like a breast. You may want to have your other breast augmented to create the size and contour you desire.

6

Bleeding & Menopause

Your estrogen level may begin to decline as early as your mid-30s and certainly through your 40s. As the estrogen level declines, your menstrual cycle may also begin to change, albeit subtly at first. You'll recognize these changes by a decrease in the amount of your menstrual flow.

Along with decreased estrogen level, you may begin to fail to ovulate every month. If you fail to ovulate (give off an egg), progesterone is not released. The lining of your uterus may not be sloughed off, and another series of problems arise. As over-growth of the inner lining of your uterus continues, it may begin to fragment and result in irregular periods or sporadic spotting.

Although your doctor may be fairly certain this bleeding is associated with not ovulating, he will take a Pap smear and perform an endometrial biopsy to confirm this diagnosis and to rule out cancer. We will discuss other causes of irregular bleeding in this chapter.

In other words, it is *common* to have changes in your menstrual period as you get older, especially as you near menopause. However, any change in your menstrual pattern is reason for checking with your doctor. Let him be the one to decide if the change in your flow should be investigated.

If the change is minor, he may elect to wait another month or so to see if this is a one-time occurrence. If it persists, he may suggest an endometrial biopsy, which is 90-percent accurate if carefully done. If the biopsy reveals no abnormality and the abnormal bleeding persists, your doctor may recommend a D&C.

- *Just what is a D&C and how is it performed?*

The letters "D&C" stand for *Dilatation and Curettage.* Dilatation means *stretching* or expansion of an opening with a dilator. This applies to your cervix or the neck (opening) of the uterus.

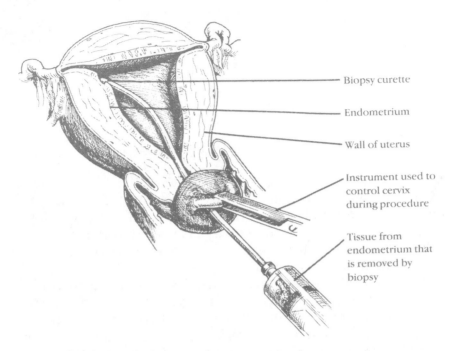

- Biopsy curette
- Endometrium
- Wall of uterus
- Instrument used to control cervix during procedure
- Tissue from endometrium that is removed by biopsy

With an endometrial biopsy, tissue can be removed easily and often painlessly from the endometrium to determine if it is normal.

Curettage means *scraping*. It refers to scraping the lining of your uterus to remove superficial tissue with a curette (scraper). This tissue is carefully collected and sent for examination in the laboratory. Refer to pages 32, 35–36 for more details.

A pathologist is a specialist who examines the tissue and determines whether it is abnormal, whether it is cancerous or benign. A D&C is *diagnostic* because it determines the cause. It is *therapeutic* in that the procedure often cures the bleeding.

Preparation and microscopic examination of the removed tissue may require 48 to 72 hours. But it is extremely accurate in ruling out cancer and helping us make a diagnosis.

The most painful part of a D&C is stretching your cervix. It may also be painful for some women to have the uterus scraped. For this reason, a D&C is performed under anesthesia.

Recovery from a D&C is rapid with no post-operative pain or discomfort from the procedure itself. Your recovery from the anesthetic is the only factor that could stop you from resuming normal activities immediately. There may be light vaginal-

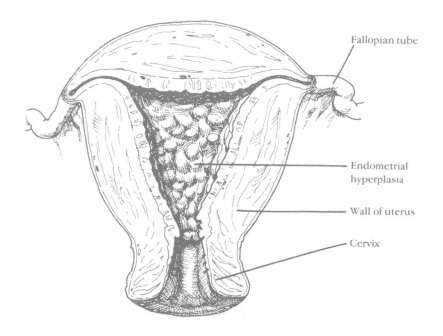

Fallopian tube

Endometrial
hyperplasia

Wall of uterus

Cervix

*Endometrial hyperplasia is an overgrowth of the lining of the uterus.
Certain types of endometrial hyperplasia may become cancerous.*

bleeding for several days after.

- *What's an endometrial biopsy? How does it differ from a D&C?*

  An endometrial biopsy is the removal of only a tiny amount of tissue from the lining of your uterus to sample it. A D&C attempts to remove *all* of the superficial lining. An endometrial biopsy can be performed in your doctor's office, using a paracervical block (local anesthesia), or in some cases without anesthesia and with only momentary discomfort.

  A long, curved metal tube or a plastic tube (pipelle), smaller than the diameter of a straw, is inserted into your uterus. Near the end of the tube, called a *biopsy curette,* is an opening with a sharp edge on its upper side. As the biopsy curette is drawn downward against the lining of your uterus, it shaves off a strip of tissue. This is sucked into the tube and sent for examination in the laboratory, just like the material removed during a D&C.

  An endometrial biopsy is about 90-percent accurate in detecting cancer. According to Dr. L. Nachtigall (1986), all endometrial cancer goes through a phase of hyperplasia (overgrowth). This is likely to be detected by endometrial biopsy. Small samples of the lining from various segments of the uterus are removed during the endometrial biopsy for analysis. Several samples may be taken during the procedure.

An endometrial biopsy is also used to determine the phase of your cycle or to determine whether or not you have ovulated. Such information may avoid the necessity for a D&C. In infertility studies or in functional bleeding (due to piling up of the lining of your uterus), an endometrial biopsy can be very useful in establishing the cause.

- *I am 48 and have had a little spotting between my menstrual periods for the last 2 months. Is this serious?*

It could be. Any change in the pattern of your menstrual periods warrants investigation. Although this spotting could be due to failure to ovulate, a polyp, or a fibroid, it could also be due to an early cancer in the lining of your uterus.

Your doctor will want to check on this spotting by performing an endometrial biopsy or a D&C. Report to him immediately. In fact, when you call for an appointment, let his receptionist know what is happening. She will undoubtedly fit you in without delay. There is more detailed information on page 25 about cancer of the uterus and its high rate of cure when detected early.

- *What is the difference between a cervical biopsy and a D&C? When I was examined a few days ago, my doctor said he took a biopsy of my cervix right while I was on the examining table. Although the biopsy was not painful, I have had some spotting since then.*

As mentioned on page 31, your cervix can be cut (biopsied), burned (cauterized), frozen or sewed without discomfort. It is painful, however, to have the opening of your cervix stretched and the uterine cavity scraped as in a D&C.

If your doctor finds a part of the cervix is irritated or looks suspicious, he will use biopsy forceps (see illustration on page 31) to "punch out" a piece of tissue from this area. The tissue will be sent to the laboratory for examination. Spotting may continue for a day or two. It is rarely severe enough to require treatment.

If the entire area around the opening to the cervix is suspicious appearing or if your Pap smear reveals abnormal cells, your doctor may evaluate your cervix with a colposcope (microscope) and take a series of punch biopsies from your cervix. Or he may

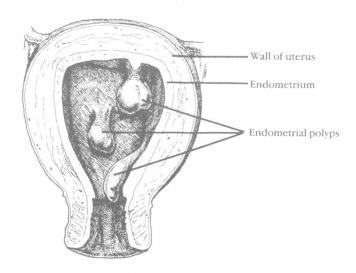

Endometrial polyps can be single or multiple and are diagnosed by D&C. Some cause bleeding, others do not.

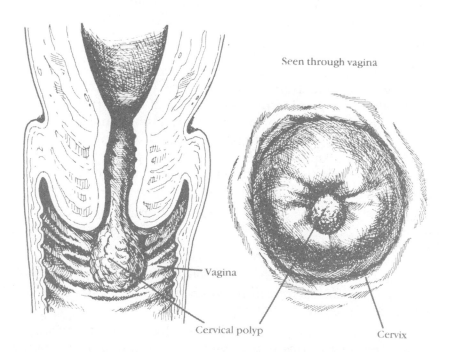

A cervical polyp hangs on a pedicle and may protrude from the cervix into the vagina. If often causes bleeding during intercourse.

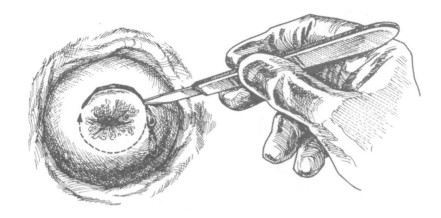

In conization, a cone of tissue is cut from the cervix with a scalpel to remove a chronic area of inflammation that does not heal.

remove a cone of tissue from your cervix. These samples will be examined to determine the extent of the disease.

- *What is conization of the cervix?*

  Under anesthesia, your doctor may remove a cone of tissue from the cervix (see illustration) and send it to the laboratory for examination. Conization removes a cone of tissue from the area surrounding the opening to the cervix. Tissue analysis should reveal where the spotting is coming from. It will also reveal the location of the suspicious cells that gave the positive Pap smear. Spotting can come from lesions on the cervix and even the vagina. Spotting is not limited to the uterus.

  Stitches are placed to control bleeding after a conization of the cervix. Your doctor has other ways to control lesser amounts of bleeding postoperatively.

- *Three months ago I practically flooded when I had my menstrual period. I have had no problems since then, but I have worried about the episode. I am 46. Do I need to do anything about this?*

  Certainly you should check with your doctor. As the supply of eggs in the ovaries decreases, your periods can and do change. Flooding is a sign you should be examined and followed closely to see if it recurs. An endometrial biopsy, in addition to a Pap smear, may be necessary. You could have an endometrial polyp

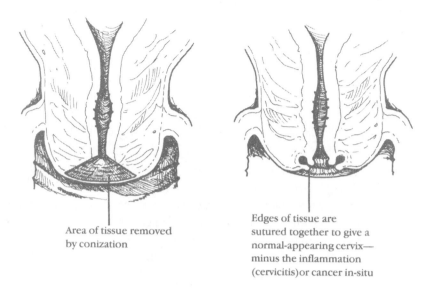

Area of tissue removed
by conization

Edges of tissue are
sutured together to give a
normal-appearing cervix—
minus the inflammation
(cervicitis) or cancer in-situ

This is the area of tissue removed by conization. Tissue edges are stitched together to give a normal-appearing cervix.

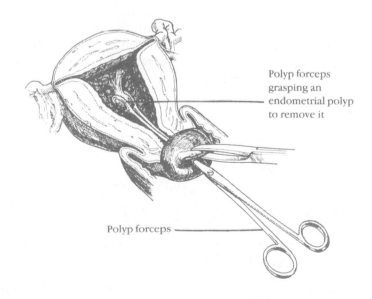

Polyp forceps
grasping an
endometrial polyp
to remove it

Polyp forceps

Endometrial polyps are removed, when possible, by grasping them with endometrial-polyp forceps.

which is an overgrowth of the uterine lining. It looks like a thick droplet of paint that is ready to drip (see illustration, page 89). This could be diagnosed by a D&C or even a hysteroscopy. This requires an instrument used to look into the cavity of the uterus, called a *hysteroscope.*

- *I am 50 and have always had regular menstrual periods. About 6 months ago I stopped altogether for 3 months. Since then I have had just a little spotting nearly every day. Is this just the tapering off before stopping permanently?*

This is not normal. You should be examined immediately to determine the cause of this spotting. It could be caused by endometrial hyperplasia (an overgrowth of the lining of your uterus due to lack of ovulation). It could also be due to an early cancer. Do not delay your visit to your doctor. Cancer of the endometrium has a high rate of cure when detected and treated early (see pages 32–34).

- *I am 49. During the last year I had everything from spotting to hemorrhage. During 2 months there was no bleeding at all. I am tired of this worry and frustration. A D&C showed no cancer.*

By taking progestogen in a cyclic fashion, it is possible to give regularity to your flow until you actually stop altogether. If hormone therapy such as this does not control the bleeding, the other possibility is a hysterectomy. A hysterectomy removes the threat of certain cancers and pregnancy.

Bleeding at the time of menopause is almost like an automobile that runs out of gas. It sputters and coughs as the gas gets low. Then it finally gives out with a dying gasp. Occasionally it is difficult to tolerate the sputtering and coughing in your menstrual periods before the final gasp occurs and bleeding stops forever. For more about endometrial hyperplasia, see page 36.

If cancer has been ruled out and you can tolerate this situation, surgery may be avoidable. The irregular pattern of bleeding will eventually end. In most instances, it can be controlled adequately and easily by hormone treatment.

- *I've had heavy menstrual periods the past several months. Examination showed large tumors in my uterus. My doctor assures me they are benign. He advised me to wait a few months to see if I go through menopause because after menopause these benign tumors will decrease in size. But I am worried about cancer. I am 48 years old.*

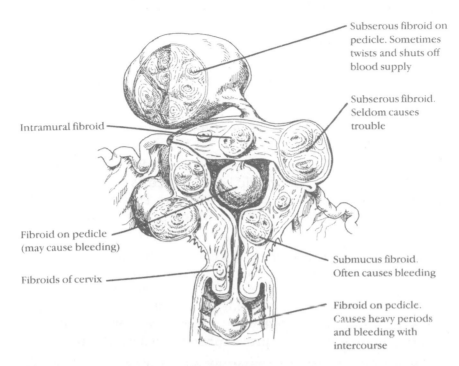

Subserous fibroid on pedicle. Sometimes twists and shuts off blood supply

Subserous fibroid. Seldom causes trouble

Intramural fibroid

Fibroid on pedicle (may cause bleeding)

Fibroids of cervix

Submucus fibroid. Often causes bleeding

Fibroid on pedicle. Causes heavy periods and bleeding with intercourse

There are many locations for fibroid tumors of the uterus. Size and location often determine symptoms.

Your doctor is right. You probably have fibroid tumors. These rarely become malignant. See illustration above. These tumors do become smaller after menopause. However, fibroid tumors may become larger if you take estrogen, the hormone that is administered to relieve hot flashes and other symptoms of menopause.

In general, fibroid tumors are not removed unless they:

1. Cause heavy bleeding unresponsive to hormonal therapy

2. Become so large as to start putting pressure on the bowel, bladder or ureters (tubes from the kidneys to the bladder)

3. Begin to grow so rapidly that malignancy is a concern; or

4. Outgrow their blood supply and cause pain.

If your doctor is following their progress carefully, fibroids can be observed with the hope they will regress in size after menopause and require no further treatment.

If your symptoms persist or progress, you may elect to have your uterus removed to rid yourself of the problem. If you are worried about cancer of the uterus because of your bleeding, your doctor can perform an endometrial biopsy or even a D&C to assure you both there is no cancer.

Cyclic progestogen, in most instances, will also control the bleeding until you reach menopause. Menopause ends all bleeding.

- *I am 45 and recently noticed some spotting after intercourse. Is this to be expected at my age?*

Spotting after intercourse is never normal. It could be a clue something is wrong. You should be examined as soon as possible to determine the cause. You could have an erosion (inflammation) of the cervix. Or it could be coming from the lining of the uterus.

To determine the cause, your doctor may not only take a Pap smear but also may biopsy or even remove a cone of tissue from the cervix. He may even perform an endometrial biopsy or a D&C. If the tests are negative for cancer of the cervix, he may cauterize (burn with a hot wire) your cervix or treat it with freezing. Both are painless procedures and foster healing.

A newer method is to treat the cervix with a laser beam. This will also remove the eroded area and permit it to heal. As mentioned earlier, your cervix can be burned, frozen, cut, sewed or lasered without much discomfort or the need for anesthesia.

Cancers of your cervix or the lining of the uterus are notably easy to treat and attended by a 95-percent 5-year cure rate if treated early. Do not wait to see if spotting after intercourse persists. Check with your doctor as soon as possible.

7

Weight Control & Menopause

Edited by Kathleen Dailey, Registered Clinical Dietitian

In certain other cultures you would be considered healthy and beautiful if you are what we label *overweight* or *plump*. Today, thin is in! Whether it is due to the fashion experts or someone else, fat, obesity—even plumpness—is judged undesirable. It may not be right, but that is the way it is. Isn't it a paradox that *thin is in* when eating is such a social event for most of us? Almost since birth, food has been the universal pacifier. Whether it was a bottle or cookie or later in life a steak dinner, food has been used to celebrate, to reward and to console.

From a health standpoint, overweight is a major risk factor. A government panel in 1985 concluded individuals who were 20-percent or more overweight were prone to premature death, arthritis, respiratory problems, gallbladder disease, adult-onset diabetes, menstrual abnormalities and high blood pressure.

In Framingham, Massachusetts (1980) where a 26-year study on most inhabitants of the town has been carefully monitored, it was found that even being 10-percent overweight caused a higher incidence of heart disease and death from all causes.

As you enter menopause, you want to do so with enthusiasm and high self-esteem. Few things dampen enthusiasm or reduce self esteem like extra unwanted pounds.

In this chapter we tell you how exercise and proper diet can help you control your weight instead of allowing it to control you.

- *How do I know if I am really overweight? Not everyone agrees on optimum weight.*

For many years the Metropolitan Life Insurance Tables have been the standard of comparison. See table on page 244. However, these tables do not consider body composition (percent body fat vs. lean weight) for recommended weights. Because muscle is more dense than fat, a more-muscular person is smaller in size than a "fatter" person, even though they are the same height and weight. Thus, your measurements, what size you wear and how your clothes fit are sometimes better guides for optimum weight.

• *I have always been reasonably thin, at least not fat, until I went through the change of life a year ago. Now I am gaining weight despite my best efforts to control the gain. Is this normal for my age? What can I do?*

At least you are not alone in North America! More than 11-million people are severely obese, which means they weigh 250 pounds or more. There wouldn't be so many overweight people if there was an easy way to lose those excess pounds!

Obesity is not due to gluttony in most cases. Obesity is a *disease* which we little understand and one we are no more successful at treating than alcoholism. One reason weight salons and fad-diet books make so much money is that we physicians have been so miserably unsuccessful in treating obesity. Fad-diet books and gimmick salons have no better success, but they do advertise well.

Many women who are gaining weight complain they are eating the same things in the same amount as they have always done— and they are correct. But they may not realize how their lifestyle has changed. But they've probably abandoned the sports they used to enjoy so enthusiastically in their teens and 20s. Perhaps they watch television more than before.

A number of us move more slowly as we enter our 30s and 40s and especially into our 50s. We conserve our energy without being aware of it. You probably eat the same, but you exercise less. You require less calories than you did when you were younger.

It's a myth that starchy foods cause us to become fat. More likely it is the fats we add to those starches (butter or margarine on breads and rolls; sour cream on baked potatoes; mayonnaise,

ề   ề   ề

The weight gain some women experience in midlife may be due to their sedentary lifestyle. While women may not eat more than they did in younger years, they exercise less.

cheese and lots of meats on sandwiches; and salad dressings).

Fat contributes 9 calories per gram as opposed to carbohydrates which contribute only 4 calories per gram. Protein foods such as dairy products, meats, poultry, cheeses and eggs are high in fat unless carefully chosen and prepared as lowfat. Fat calories should contribute less than 30% of the day's total calories. This should be less than 20% for losing weight. Carbohydrates can supply over 50% of the day's total calories. These should principally come from whole-grain breads and cereals; starches, fruits and vegetables.

Unless you are more than 20-percent overweight, the simple changes listed above will probably do it for you without resorting to a low-calorie diet. If you require more discipline than this to lose weight, simply decrease your fat calories rather than following some crash diet or expensive weight-loss plan.

- *I have never had a weight problem before. In fact, I have never had to concern myself with weight-control in my life. But since my 40th birthday I have steadily put on weight. When will it stop? Is this part of my beginning menopause?*

As a woman's body prepares for menopause, there is a gradual decline in estrogen production that begins in the mid-30s. Even though thyroid testing cannot now prove it, the metabolism (rate at which your body converts calories into energy) appears to slow down. Women who never had a weight problem find pounds begin to creep on as they near menopause. Maintaining or losing weight is possible, but it will require more exercise and a change in one's eating habits to focus on lowfat eating.

- *Are you opposed to all these diet and exercise spas?*

Absolutely not! Many women have shed unwanted pounds through various programs. But they are expensive and often time-consuming. More importantly, if you fail to change your eating habits (*behavior modification*) as part of any of these programs, you will regain your lost pounds just as soon as you discontinue the program.

Advantages of these programs are they require you to check with them often. Many offer sociability with others who share the same problems. Or, you can follow the diet and exercise plans recommended by the American Heart Association and accomplish the same goals with no expense.

We caution you to avoid all crash diets and fad-diet books with their strange ideas. Most are conceived by someone who knows little if anything about sensible nutrition. Calories can be cut without sacrificing good sense and the balanced diet you need.

It's possible to maintain the same weight in midlife you had in your 20s, but it will be more difficult as years go by. If it means that much to you and if you are willing to make the effort, you can do it by lowfat eating, combined with a sensible exercise program. Only you can decide if this is what you want.

Rather than wasting your time, money and effort on fat farms, fad diets and reducing salons, spend your effort in eliminating some of the other high-risk factors besides obesity that threaten your health and life. These include cigarette smoking, high blood pressure and high cholesterol levels.

- *How successful is the stapling operation?*

In general, you will not be accepted for a stapling operation on your stomach unless you are under 50 years old, more than 100-pounds overweight and have tried seriously to lose weight and have failed. The operation is successful if you are committed to losing weight.

In a stapling procedure, staples are placed across your stomach so that only a 2-ounce pouch remains to serve as your stomach. The pouch exit is also stapled. The result is a 2-ounce stomach which is quickly filled while the tiny exit permits food to leave the pouch slowly and only if the food is pureed.

If you force-feed yourself, it's possible to break the stapling, thus enlarging the stomach to its former size. When this happens, you will regain your excess weight. Because obesity is a potentially life-threatening disease, many physicians recommend their obese patients have a stapling operation if they meet the above standards. In many overweighters, this operation has proved lifesaving, and has restored their self-esteem as it restored their desired body contour.

- *Why is it the harder I try, the more difficult it becomes to lose weight? I am amazed at how only a few calories can keep my body going without giving up more weight.*

Your body is so smart it adjusts to a lower caloric intake. The more you cut down on your calories, the more efficient your body becomes. Dramatically decreasing caloric intake forces the body to take the energy it needs by breaking down muscle mass, not stored fat. This increases the body-fat percent. Regular physical exercise stimulates metabolism and helps you maintain lean tissue. If you combine exercise with your lowfat diet, you will eventually lose weight.

- *Is it true I should leave alcohol alone if I am dieting?*

Alcohol contains no nutritional benefits and is high in calories. If alcohol is consumed on a daily or regular basis, weight-loss efforts may be slowed.

- *I agree amphetamines should not be used for dieting. In fact, I understand because of their addicting effect, it is illegal to prescribe them for dieting. However, doctors seem hesitant about prescribing the pills that are not addicting. Why?*

Doctors don't have to prescribe these diet pills because they are available over-the-counter without prescription. They have a mild appetite-suppressing effect, but with several disadvantages. Package inserts for phenylpropanolamine warn against its use when high blood pressure, coronary heart disease, heart irregularities, diabetes and thyroid disease are present.

If you lose weight while taking the pills and then discontinue them, what have you accomplished if you turn right around and regain the weight? And if you are one of the unfortunate patients who develops a brain hemorrhage or some other serious complication, is it worth the risk? Only if you are willing to change your diet and your activity (called *behavior modification*), will you be able to lose weight and keep it off.

This must be a lifetime commitment or you will soon regain the weight you have lost and a little bit more.

- *I don't mind getting older, but I do mind getting fatter. The claims of these weight-control groups sound enticing. Because I have tried everything else, I feel I might as well give them a chance.*

Before you enroll in one of these programs, remember they are expensive and their results do not last unless you change your lifestyle at the same time.

In certain programs, you are quoted a high fee to be paid up front. You will then have "analyses" of your hair, nails, body secretions, hormones and what they call *cytotoxic testing*.

Some salons could hand you a standard form report on these tests because nearly all the results are the same for every participant. Most will show you are allergic to almost everything, and you have been eating all wrong. They'll tell you your body is lacking several ingredients—available from this group at a high price.

You will soon be eating right out of their hands and paying handsomely. If you are fortunate enough to lose some weight, you'll regain it within a short time after you stop the program.

Some programs have adequate and sound nutritional programs with little or no fanfare. You have to be the judge. Some are time-tested and reliable. Sound programs recommend a diet which is lower in fat, does not eliminate any food groups (i.e., dairy or starches) and emphasizes regular physical activity. Caloric intake should not be less than 1,000 calories per day without monitoring by a physician.

- *I heard my weight depends to a great extent upon how many fat cells I have and I can do nothing about them. Is this true?*

Yes, to a degree. If you were a fat child, you are likely to be a fat adult because of the many fat cells you developed while a child. These fat cells are always on the prowl to store fat if you allow yourself any extra calories. Over a period of time you can overcome this proneness to store extra fat, but it will not be easy.

- *How valuable is fish oil or a fish-oil pill?*

Fish oil contains a special polyunsaturated fatty acid called *Omega-3*, which the fish get from certain cold-water plants. Omega-3 will reduce blood clotting, prevent hardening of your arteries, lessen your chance of heart attack due to a clot in the coronary (heart) arteries, lower total cholesterol and triglyceride, and raise desirable HDL (high-density lipoprotein) cholesterol.

- *If fish oil is so marvelous, why shouldn't everyone take it?*

Fish oil decreases the clotting ability of your blood, thereby increasing the risk of a hemorrhagic type of stroke. This effect increases danger in an accident or during surgery when it is important for your blood to clot normally. Much more research must be done on fish oil.

Fish oil may contain pesticides if made from fish livers, because this is where such toxins are concentrated. Pesticides may tend to cause malignancies. Cod-liver oil is especially rich in vitamins A and D, which can be toxic in high doses.

Fish oil taken over a long period of time may result in a vitamin-E deficiency. We are not sure what dose of Omega-3 is needed, so we suggest you eat fish rather than taking the oil capsules.

- *I am confused about various oils for eating and cooking. Can you give us some simple guidelines?*

Because vegetable oils have become an important part of American eating habits, let us list a few things you might want to know:

1. All oils are simply fat in liquid form.

2. No vegetable oil contains cholesterol. Cholesterol is found only in animal products.

3. No vegetable oil is 100-percent polyunsaturated or monounsaturated. Corn, soybean, safflower and other kinds of oil all contain some saturated fatty acids. But they are certainly better than animal fats such as lard. Canola oil is the most desirable of these oils.

4. Avoid coconut and palm-kernel oil. Although these are often used because of their long shelf-life, they are highly saturated.

5. Avoid foods containing hydrogenated oils, because hydrogenation makes fat far more saturated.

6. Heat cooking oil before adding food. The food will cook faster and absorb less oil.

7. Stir-fried vegetables and meat cook faster and with less oil.

8. Use non-stick pans to avoid adding oils.

9. A brush lets you coat a pan with less oil, or use a spray-on vegetable oil.

10. Make your own salad dressing using two parts highly unsaturated oil to one part vinegar or lemon juice. Add fresh or dried herbs or spices and mustard.

11. Monounsaturated fatty acids found in olive oil and canola oil have been identified as "protectors" of HDL (the "good" cholesterol). These oils do not raise HDL, but prevent its fall. Diets containing high levels of polyunsaturated fatty acids caused HDL to fall. Therefore, canola and olive oils are the most desirable in the diet.

- *Everyone is eating and drinking low-calorie foods, nearly all of which contain NutraSweet® or Equal®. How safe is this? Will it really help me keep down the calories?*

NutraSweet® is the trade name for aspartame. It's used in many products, principally diet drinks, desserts and ice cream. Aspartame is 180 to 200 times as sweet as sugar. That is why you get by with so few calories when you eat and drink "sugarless" foods.

Aspartame does not encourage tooth decay as sugar does. It does not cause a bitter aftertaste as some sugar substitutes do. To date, aspartame is not associated with cancer.

- *Because nothing is perfect, what are the disadvantages of NutraSweet®?*

Among other things, some people are allergic to it and develop swelling of their larynx (voice box). It has been accused, but not convicted, of causing seizures in children. It may be toxic in high doses. For example, don't allow a child to drink a 2-liter bottle of diet drink.

Aspartame may have irreversible and toxic effects on a fetal brain. Pregnant women, nursing mothers and infants under 6 months should avoid it.

There's no evidence that drinking diet soft drinks or eating artificially sweetened foods will help anyone to lose weight.

- *Breakfast is the easiest meal for me to skip. I have never felt any ill effect from missing it. I feel, at 50, I need all the help I can get to keep calories down. Am I doing the right thing?*

You are just one of an estimated 24 percent of the adult population who skip breakfast. The truth is many people who eat breakfast, eat an unhealthy one consisting of bacon, eggs, doughnuts, Danish, sugary cereals, pancakes smothered in syrup and on and on.

What kind of breakfast should you eat? If you eat the kind described above, you might be better off to skip it. If you are going to eat breakfast, consider the following:

Bagels. Plain bagels are recommended because they contain high-protein flour and little fat. Avoid egg bagels.

Bread. The most nutritious bread is 100-percent whole-wheat or whole-grain bread. Look for breads made with little or no shortening, oils or butter—such as bagels, sourdough bread and breads by special bakeries. The essential item to look for is the quantity of fat per bagel or slice of bread. It should be 3 grams or less.

Butter. For cooking, substitute a non-stick pan coated with vegetable oil. For spreading, substitute peanut butter, apple butter or all-fruit spreads containing little or no sugar.

Cottage or ricotta cheese. These are a nice change for breakfast. Cottage cheese with fresh fruit is satisfying.

Croissants. Avoid on a daily basis because they contain butter, sugar, saturated fat, cholesterol and lots of calories.

Eggs. Use more egg whites and less yolk to cut down on cholesterol. Or, use an egg substitute.

Fast foods. Most are fried and loaded with fat and sodium. They are low in fiber and high in calories.

High-fiber foods. Make certain they are high-fiber and not coated with sugar, honey or salt as in granola.

Margarine. Use a soft variety with twice as much polyunsaturate. A diet margarine contains more water and air and only half the calories. Stick margarine contains more saturated fat.

Milk. Substitute lowfat or skim milk. Fruit added to milk makes it more palatable, but most people learn to tolerate nonfat (skim) or lowfat milk—or even substitute water as a beverage. Consider lowfat buttermilk.

Pancakes. Excellent if made from whole-wheat flour, cooked with minimum oil in a non-stick pan and served with fruit, applesauce or juice concentrate instead of syrup.

Vitamins and minerals. These do not have to be added if your diet is well-balanced. If you are following a restricted-calorie diet (less than 1200 calories per day), then a daily multivitamin--mineral supplement (one providing no more than 100% of the recommended daily allowances—RDAs) is recommended.

Yogurt. Plain nonfat or lowfat yogurt can be substituted for whipped cream, dairy sour cream and cream cheeses.

- *Do you agree every one has a "set point" and it is difficult to gain or lose more than 10 to 15 pounds from this set point?*

This is true for most people. You may have noticed this yourself. But persistent overeating can raise your set point. By determined, yet sensible eating, plus a regular physical-exercise program, you can also lower your set point. Realize it will take considerable time and effort. Such a change does not come overnight.

- *I have gained weight mostly around my hips and in my breasts since my menopause. Now at 58, I am determined to lose this weight. What do you suggest?*

First, try a lowfat diet consisting mostly of complex carbohydrates (potatoes, bread, rice, whole grains, fruits and vegetables) without the cream, sugar and butter. If you are successful at losing weight in all areas but your hips or your breasts, you may want to consider subcutaneous suction lipectomy or reduction mammaplasty as a last resort, see pages 200–204 for more information.

Lowfat, high complex-carbohydrate diets should help you lose weight, especially if you combine them with an exercise program. See page 119.

- *Does coffee really increase the risk of heart disease?*

This debate began about 15 years ago when it was claimed coffee did indeed increase the risk of heart disease. Then it was discovered many of those in the study were also smokers. Coffee seemed vindicated. Needless to say, the 80 percent of all North Americans who drink coffee were relieved.

Then in 1984, a study of 2,000 men, aged 40 to 56, showed non-smoking men who drink more than 6 cups of coffee daily have twice as much coronary heart disease as those who drink less. Research by S. Mathias and others (1985) has shown this amount of coffee can raise cholesterol levels by as much as 14 percent. This is a possible reason for the increased number of cases of coronary-artery disease.

Certainly other factors contribute to coronary-artery disease, such as obesity, Type-A personality, sedentary lifestyle and high cholesterol intake. All these factors could influence these figures. If you drink coffee, be moderate. Two cups of coffee might be safer than 6! Better yet, consider decaffeinated coffees and teas.

- *I have never been an exerciser. But I must admit I have failed to control my weight by dieting. How important is exercise in weight control?*

If you decrease your total calories sufficiently, you will lose weight. You can also lose weight with exercise alone, assuming the total calories are not unreasonably high. But it's difficult.

Ideally you should combine exercise with a decrease in calories. Not only will you find it much easier to lose weight, but it will be more successful and faster. Read page 119 to find out how to begin exercises. Follow the suggestions in this chapter concerning elimination of desserts, second helpings and snacks. You may find this is all you need to do to lose your extra pounds.

One important precaution: If you decide to walk or jog, take a companion—preferably a dog—for protection.

- *I have heard and read so much about using salt, sugar and fats in my cooking. Are they really that bad?*

We are accustomed to all three of these flavors in our foods. But nearly the whole population would benefit from a reduction in their use. Here are a few suggestions about acceptable substitutes:

In place of	Substitute
Salt	Single or mixed herbs: basil, cilantro, dill, marjoram, oregano, rosemary, thyme. Lemon juice, lime juice or both.
Sugar	Half the amount, sugar substitute, or use concentrated fruit juices.
Whole milk, cream, dairy sour cream	Skim milk, lowfat or nonfat yogurt, nonfat cottage cheese pureed in a blender with a little lemon juice.
Whole egg	2 egg whites, or use an egg substitute.
Butter and fats	Soft margarine or vegetable oil for shortening. Use a non-stick pan for cooking and/or use a vegetable-base non-stick spray such as Pam®. Use herbs (see Salt, above) and lemon or lime juice as seasoning for vegetables. Trim fat from meat before cooking. Remove poultry skin before cooking or eating.
Oil-based marinades	Herb-flavored vinegar, red or white wine, lemon juice, low-salt broth, low-salt soy sauce.
Salad dressing	Use vinegar and oil plus spices and herbs.
Ice cream	Nonfat frozen yogurt, sherbet, ice milk or sorbet.
Cream cheese	Yogurt cheese or nonfat yogurt and cottage cheese combined.
Soft drinks	Unsweetened fruit juices, flavored bottled or carbonated water.
Food preparation	Bake, broil, microwave or steam foods whenever possible, Avoid frying.

8

Partners & Menopause

Because you have now reached the point in your life where pregnancy is a closed chapter, it may be a good time to renew or at least fortify the relationship between you and your partner. Your sexual relationship may need some revitalization. At least it deserves a second look.

To your dismay, you may find the man in your life is going through some emotional as well as physical changes of his own. He may not want to discuss these changes with you. In his mind, they often pose themselves more as challenges than changes. It is important you talk things over. You may have to be the tactful one to bring up the subject of your relationship.

One of the greatest tests of your skill in communication may be to initiate a discussion of sensitive midlife problems in such a way they neither imply nor even suggest a challenge to your partner's self-esteem. Avoid words like "never" and "always" in such phrases as "You *always* do this," "You *never* do that," or "you *think* this or that." Try, "Is there any way in which I might improve our relationship?" Or, "Do you feel I am responsive to your feelings?"

If you can get him talking about it, you have already reached an important milestone in preparing both of you for a good relationship during your menopause and what can be the golden years that follow. This certainly is not the time for put-downs or pressures for either partner.

Unfortunately sexual prowess has wrongfully become a sign of *machismo* for many men. By contrast, impotence is such a devastating experience, most men avoid even mentioning the subject—though they definitely desire relief for such a problem. This is the area in which an understanding wife can do more than anyone else (including a sex counselor) to help him deal with and usually overcome the problem.

- *How common is impotence in men?*

It's estimated there are about 10-million impotent men in the United States. We don't know how reliable that figure is, because men are reluctant to talk about the subject—especially if *they* have the problem.

In recent years, this subject is being discussed openly in both public and medical forums. Entire television programs have been devoted to the subject. We are learning more about impotence and its causes. Hope for better treatment seems justified.

- *What causes impotence in men?*

At one time the problem was turned over to psychiatrists, because it was assumed impotence was emotional and undoubtedly due to some psychological hang-up. We are now finding many cases of impotence are due to physical, organic disorders, or medications. Many of these causes can be relieved.

Male erection seems simple enough to those who have no problem with it. Male arousal, erection and ejaculation are complicated processes that can run into difficulty anywhere between the thought processes in the brain and the end result in the penis.

First of all, the psyche must be such that the brain gives the nerve the go-ahead. Then glandular mechanisms in the body must allow the nerve stimulus to act on the arteries that flow to the penis. These penile arteries must be healthy enough to deliver up to 7 times the usual amount of blood to the penis—enough to stiffen it. Next, ejaculation and orgasm must be permitted to complete themselves without interference.

Countless diseases, medications, functional disorders and emotional problems can intercede anywhere along the way to prevent the desired end-result. Let's list a few of these common deterrents to normal functioning:

Organic Diseases

1. Heart disease. In general, if a man can climb two flights of stairs, intercourse will not hurt him. His heart disease is not likely to keep him from performing. But his anxiety about his heart disease or your own anxiety as his partner may make him impotent, especially after a heart attack or after heart surgery.

2. Diabetes. Diabetes can interfere with blood supply to the penis and may narrow the blood vessels enough to prevent erection. Exercise and meticulous control of the diabetes will minimize this and other side effects.

3 . Hypothyroidism. The fatigue that goes along with hypothyroidism may interfere with sexual function, but the condition can be treated medically.

4. High blood pressure. High blood pressure of long-standing can cause narrowing of the blood vessels to the penis, thus preventing erection.

Emotional Factors

1. Anxiety. Worry about financial or other conditions, including worry about not being able to perform when a man has once failed, can be a serious factor. You can help your mate overcome this fear and worry by patience, assurance and by taking plenty of time to talk when you make love. Do not make intercourse, penetration or ejaculation a must. Your partner cannot *will* an erection anyway. The more a man worries about failing to perform, the more likely he is to fail. In general, if a man has erections during his sleep, he will still be able to have them when awake if worry, fatigue and fear of failure are eliminated.

2. Depression. Depression can cause impotence, but you must be aware antidepressant drugs may also cause impotence.

Medicines

More than 75 medicines list "possible impotence" as one of their side effects. Some common offenders are tranquilizers, diuretics, beta-blocker drugs, Aldomet®, Ismelin® and Tagamet®.

Certainly you should check with your doctor to see if the medicine your husband is taking might have impotence as a side effect. Have your husband ask the pharmacist for a copy of the package insert for each of the drugs he is taking. Read it to see if impotence is a possible side effect.

Drugs

Alcohol in small amounts might "loosen up" your husband so he desires intercourse. But too much alcohol will cause him to fall on his face as far as performing when he makes love.

There is even some evidence that heavy smoking narrows the blood vessels in the penis enough to interfere with erection. Cocaine and other drugs do not heighten sexual response. They lessen sensation and may cause complete impotence.

Cancer of the Prostate

Whether due to cancer or not, surgical removal or resection of the prostate gland may cause impotence. In certain cases, resection (reaming of the prostate) may cause your partner's ejaculate to be regurgitated into his bladder rather than ejected from the penis. This does not interfere with erection or orgasm.

- *My husband and I are both 45. Recently he has begun to gain weight, slack off on exercise, lose motivation and even the desire for sex. This seems unusual for someone who has always been sexually active.*

Your husband may be depressed. Depression is one of the most common and most overlooked illnesses. Because depression can be devastating, even to the point of suicide, you should insist he seek medical help.

Depression is also one of the most treatable conditions with a host of effective antidepressant medicines available. As mentioned, you should realize antidepressant drugs may also cause your partner's impotence.

As far as your husband's excess weight gain is concerned, you can be extremely helpful, because you determine, to a great extent, what he eats. Cut down on the salt you add to your cooking. Cook foods that contain smaller amounts of salt and less saturated fats. Avoid ham, bacon and highly salted foods. Many people with high blood pressure find their blood pressure returns to normal when they eliminate salt from their diet.

Substitute skim milk in place of whole milk. This may be easier if you start with 1-percent milk. Don't buy ice cream, cookies, pastries and desserts in general. If you have carrot strips or celery sticks on ice available in your refrigerator, your husband may substitute these for higher-calorie sweets. Fruits, dried or fresh, are also excellent snacks.

Beer is fattening. Diet drinks may help, but encourage your partner to drink more water or even fruit juices.

Suggest the two of you begin walking together, gradually increasing the distance and the pace. It can become a delightful exercise both of you will look forward to after your evening dinner or even early in the morning.

- *Do men go through a sort of menopause of their own?*

Many men go through a "midlife crisis," most often between the ages of 40 to 45. They may begin to doubt their sexual capabilities, worry about advancing age, the possible loss of virility and their attractiveness to the opposite sex. Depression and even panic are not unusual.

Night sweats are common. Fatigue or even hyperactivity are unpredictable. Depression may cause some loss of libido. But it can also cause some men to be sexually hyperactive in an effort to prove to themselves they are still sexually potent.

If you will be patient, tolerant and understanding, you can help your partner through this difficult period, thus saving your relationship and his future. Some men seek extramarital affairs during this time to reassure themselves of their virility.

We mention this not to condone their erratic behavior but to help you understand it. If your husband and you can survive the insecurity and frustration of this period of his life, your marriage will undoubtedly come out of the ordeal stronger than ever.

- *Is the so-called "male menopause" due to a lack of testosterone?*

It is true the level of testosterone (male sex hormone) declines slightly as men become older. But the so-called "male menopause," if it exists, is thought to be a social and emotional change, rather than one based upon any hormone change. After a man has reached the goals he set for himself, whether financial, educational, political or social, where does he go? Does he set new goals? Has he lost his challenges? Is he now over the hill? Is it downhill from here on out? Perhaps these goals have not been reached and there is a pervading sense of disappointment, inadequacy and even anxiety.

These are some of the questions that may plague your husband as he enters midlife. If you can, sense some of his feelings and fears: competition with younger men and a possible loss of youth and virility. By giving him emotional and physical support you may help him cope with his "midlife crisis" and enter the proverbial gate to the golden years the two of you have ahead of you.

ෙ   ෙ   ෙ

Men often have a tendency to gain weight in midlife for the same reason women do—a sedentary, no-exercise lifestyle.

- *My husband, at 50, has begun having night sweats. At times he wakes up soaking wet in the middle of the night for no apparent reason. Are these sweats comparable to hot flashes in women?*

No one has ever been able to link these night sweats to any hormonal change. But neither has anyone offered any rational explanation for them. They do not seem to be harmful in any way, especially if they do not disturb his sleep (or yours) too much. Most men can turn over and go back to sleep again, apparently none the worse for the experience.

- *My husband is 54 and has complained lately that my vagina is too loose for satisfactory intercourse. This has never been a problem before. Could it be his fault rather than mine?*

It is common for the muscles of your vagina to become somewhat relaxed during menopause and thereafter, possibly due to the loss of estrogen. Kegel exercises will help to strengthen these muscles. (See page 189.) It is also possible the muscles in your pelvic floor are stretched enough so you require a vaginal repair.

Generally speaking, if you require tightening of the muscles of your pelvic floor to improve intercourse, you usually have some relaxation of the support under your bladder and over your rectum. If you have difficulty controlling your urine when you strain, cough or sneeze or if you have terminal constipation (difficulty expelling the stool from the terminal part of your rectum), you may need a complete repair of all of these tissues. Check with your doctor to see if an A&P repair is necessary.

Another reason your husband has more difficulty reaching an orgasm may be due to *his* age, yet he wrongly blames you and the condition of your vagina. Talk things over, take a longer time for stimulation and arousal. Don't feel pressured during intercourse. Simply communicating better will help you meet each other's needs and may solve the problem for both of you.

- *I am 48, single and have many boy friends. I look younger than my age and lead an active sex life. For many years I have taken the birth-control pill but wonder about the upcoming menopause. I am still having normal, regular menstrual periods. How do I know when to stop taking my pills? I am having a few hot flashes but not enough to worry about.*

If you are a smoker, we don't recommend birth-control pills because of the possibility of blood clots. Healthy, non-smoking women may take the low-dose birth-control pills until they are menopausal.[1] A condom is recommended as a means of birth control and as protection from sexually transmitted diseases when several partners are involved.

If you continue to take the pill, your menstrual periods will also continue. An FSH blood test tells whether you are in menopause.

If your FSH blood test is elevated, you can discontinue all birth control and feel safe from the threat of pregnancy. Have your boyfriends use condoms anyway if you want to be sure you will not contract sexually transmitted diseases such as herpes or AIDS.

- *I am 52. For the first time in our married life, my husband complains our lovemaking is uncomfortable for him. He feels I am too dry. Frankly, I have a similar complaint. Intercourse is becoming more painful each time we make love. At times it breaks the tissues, and I have even had some bleeding after intercourse. Is this part of menopause?*

When your body fails to secrete sufficient estrogen, your genital tissues become thinner and you have less vaginal secretion. You also fail to secrete more fluid when you become aroused.

Vaginal Hygiene

1. As your vaginal secretions diminish during midlife, you may have to use a vaginal lubricant such as Replens®, H-R®, K-Y® or Lubafax® lubricating jelly to relieve the dryness during intercourse.

2. You may need ERT. See page 151 for information on estrogen-replacement therapy. If dryness of your vagina is a problem, estrogen vaginal cream used daily for 2 to 4 weeks, then 2 to 3 times each week will take care of the problem.

- *I am 51 and stopped having my menstrual periods 2 years ago. Ever since I stopped menstruating, my husband has been impotent. He is as frustrated as I am. Where should we seek help?*

Many cases of impotence can be helped. Some are emotional, some are due to organic problems. But most can be solved, allowing his impotence to clear up. Here are some suggestions:

1. Review with your doctor the medications your husband is taking to see if any of them cause impotence. Read the package

---

1   Mischell, D.R. "Contraceptive Practices in Older Women." *Obstetrics and Gynecology Audio Digest.* Oct. 5, 1990. 37, 19.

insert for each of the drugs he is taking to see if impotence is listed as a side effect.

2. Suggest your husband have a physical examination to eliminate the possibility that certain diseases, such as prostatitis and diabetes, are causing his impotence.

3. Too much alcohol or certain drugs can cause impotence.

4. Talk with your doctor about the possibility of an emotional cause for his impotence.

5. As a medical last resort, his doctor may prescribe testosterone. In general, this male hormone helps only if his level of hormone is low. This ordinarily would not occur until your husband reaches his 70s or 80s. Continued use of testosterone can also cause enlargement of his prostate gland.

6. Finally, there are permanent rigid implants and inflatable implants for insertion in the penis to help obtain erection. Talk to your doctor and he can direct you to those specialists who have had experience with these devices.

- *Is it all right for a woman to take douches? I feel unclean when I don't take a douche and feel more comfortable having sex after one.*

This is often a matter of personal hygiene. Although your vagina has a method of cleansing itself by a constant flow of discharge, this varies in different women. A vinegar douche will often relieve itching, just as some of the commercial douches will. If a douche bag is used, it must be kept clean and free of infection.

A douche can be harmful if it destroys normal vaginal bacteria or if it produces dryness in you. But to rule out vaginal douching entirely would be to say all women are the same. Follow your individual preference.

Here are a few recommendations concerning your vagina:

1. Cotton panties are preferable if you are having any problems with itching, discharge or irritation. Cotton allows ventilation, is more absorbent and often easier to wash.

2. If you experience discomfort with intercourse, first try lubrication. Replens®, H-R®, K-Y® or Lubafax® lubricating jellies are preferable to petroleum jelly.

3. Nighttime provides an opportunity to go without underpants and give the vagina a chance to air out.

4. Many women have found sanitary pads permit an infection

or irritation to clear up, one that might have been perpetuated by internal tampons. If tampons are used, change each time you go to the bathroom and use only pads at night.

5. Cleanliness is admirable, but you can be too meticulous in using soaps that remove the normal, protective body oils. Bubble baths are especially severe on natural body oils.

6. If your doctor gives you penicillin or other antibiotics for some infection such as a sore throat, these antibiotics may also kill the protective bacteria in your vagina, thus permitting a yeast infection. If you have this problem, inform your doctor so he can give you an antifungal antibiotic along with the antibacterial medicine.

7. Hot tubs can cause infections because the chlorine evaporates, leaving the water vulnerable to infection. Even herpes can be conveyed in this manner.

8. If you have repeated yeast infections, it is important that you be checked for diabetes. Several of our diabetic patients have first been suspected and subsequently diagnosed because they had repeated vaginal yeast infections.

9. Because of the danger of AIDS infections and other sexually transmitted disease, insist that your sex partner use a condom if you do not know for sure he is free of infection. Remember you are exposed to any infection any of his sex partners may have had.

❧ ❧ ❧

Some men face a "mid-life crisis" that is more challenging to them than menopause is to women.

9

Fitness & Menopause

A woman loses both muscle mass and muscle strength and has an increase in total body fat as she ages. An exercise program that includes both aerobic and resistance training may prevent or relieve some of the problems encountered with aging. These include muscle weakness, age-related increases in body fat, cardiovascular disease, osteoporosis and depression. Aerobic exercises are done continuously at a sustained elevated heart rate and can include running, walking and cycling. Resistance training to strengthen muscles should be initiated under supervision of a physical therapist or exercise physiologist, and can then be continued into later life once a woman feels comfortable and confident in doing it on her own.

Inactivity—not hormonal change—is the most common cause of weight gain. Fat is lost much more effectively by exercising than by dieting. Aerobic exercise promotes loss of abdominal fat more readily than fat at other sites. Exercise promotes loss of fat by increasing the energy one uses, increasing the metabolic rate and reducing the fat on the abdomen and other sites. The only way to increase lean body mass (muscle-to-fat ratio) is by exercising.[1]

- *Is it wise to keep jogging as I get older? I have heard it will eventually wear out my knee joints. Is this true? I am 51 and have jogged for 10 years.*

Moderate jogging (a mile or two—avoid marathons) will not wear out your knees if they are healthy to begin with. Most studies show walking, jogging and running actually strengthen your muscles, tendons and bones. If you should begin to have pain in your knees, slow down, shorten the distance and time or

1 Shangold, M.M. "Exercises in the Menopausal Woman." *Obstetrics and Gynecology.* 1990. 75:53S-58S.

replace jogging with cycling, walking, swimming or some other less-demanding activity for a while.

Older women who have not jogged before should not take it up for the first time in their lives without seeing their physician and receiving instructions on what form of exercise is best for them. Your physician can also provide information on resistance training to strengthen weak muscles. When a jogger's foot strikes the ground it lands with three times the body weight. This force often injures older bones, tendons, ligaments, joints and muscles, according to Dr. Mona Shangold (1987).

- *What are low-impact aerobics?*

Some women exchange the bouncing type of aerobics for low-impact aerobics designed to protect your knees, ankles and hips. During the non-bounce, low-impact aerobics, one foot is always kept in contact with the floor. As a result, these exercises consist principally of movements of your upper body.

Low impact does not mean low intensity, but it does involve low kicks rather than high ones. It consists of fast-paced steps, often exaggerated—such as raising the knees higher, side-to-side movements and vigorous lunges. Low-impact aerobics are particularly designed for people who have foot deformities, poor aerobic form and low strength levels. But they can be enjoyable for almost everyone.

Because low-impact aerobics place emphasis upon back movements, they may not agree with your tender back unless you are gradually able to strengthen the muscles and general support of your back. Menopausal women should not try to keep up with women in their 20s. They should also be careful about knee kicks and lunges that are too vigorous.

Low-impact aerobics may be just the type of exercise many menopausal women will tolerate best.

- *I have not engaged in sports since I was in high school and I never exercise. But I would like to start, even though I am 50. How do you*

ê•   ê•   ê•

Some women find their knees will not tolerate jogging or even extensive walking. For them, swimming may be the answer.

suggest I go about it?

First of all, you should have a physical examination in which your doctor determines whether or not you should exercise. Your physician can also recommend whether or not there are any limitations or restrictions that should be placed upon you. If you pass your physical examination, you might begin with walking as your first exercise. Those who cannot walk because of bad feet, knees or hips may have to take up swimming or bicycling.

Some women become winded even when going up one flight of stairs or walking 100 yards. At any rate, get started. Don't try to set a record in distance or speed the first time out. Remember whatever distance you walk *from* your home, you have to *return*. Begin with a short distance and walk slowly.

Don't try to keep up with anyone else. Do what you can do without becoming winded. Be consistent and try to walk every day, increasing the distance very gradually each time. As you walk a little farther each day, increase your speed, however slightly. You will be surprised how rapidly you can increase both speed and distance once you get into walking.

You may decide to limit your exercise to walking. Many studies have indicated fast walking can be as beneficial as jogging. Once you reach the mile mark, whether walking or jogging, you will find you get your second wind and can go considerably farther without difficulty.

If you are swimming, first try one pool length, then a full lap. Increase the distance every few days. You'll find your second wind, just as you did with walking and jogging. You are now on your way and merely need to be sure you continue exercising on a regular basis.

A good rule to follow is this: Exercise at least 3 or 4 times a week for at least 20 to 30 minutes, fast enough to maintain your heart rate at 75 percent of maximum. Your maximum heart rate is determined by subtracting your age from 220. For instance, if you are 50, your maximum heart rate should be 220 - 50 = 170 beats per minute. Then take 75 percent of 170 and you have 127 beats per minute. Count your pulse for 15 seconds and multiply by 4 to get the rate per minute.

- *I am simply not the exercising type. Is it really necessary for me to exercise vigorously after menopause?*

It may be just as unwise to force yourself to exercise as to avoid exercise. Look for moderation in exercising. Begin with short, slow walks to interesting areas—even to shopping malls. You may want to drive to different areas, then walk around these areas.

You will improve your quality of life and self-sufficiency into later life by developing and maintaining a regular exercise program.

A study by Dr. Alvar Svanborg, Chairman of Geriatric and Long-Term-Care Medicine at the University of Gothenburg in Sweden showed ,"Even at the age of 81, we can improve physical performance by training." At age 70, 95 percent of the active elderly had no advanced handicap. Our advice is to find an exercise that you enjoy. But do not let yourself deteriorate because of a lack of interest in exercising.

- *I have heard walking, if it becomes a regular part of your routine, will prolong life. Is this true?*

The New England Journal of Medicine reported one study suggesting significantly longer life if you walk an average of 9 miles a week. Other studies demonstrated that walking is good for nearly everyone, including those who are not into exercise.

A study at Western New Mexico University showed treadmill walking improved cardiovascular fitness and increased percentage of lean body mass at the expense of fat cells in both premenopausal and postmenopausal women. Postmenopausal women had an additional benefit because as a weight-bearing exercise, walking helped slow the process of osteoporosis.

Further studies at the University of Louisville School of Medicine showed brisk walking (about 3-1/2 miles per hour) produced definite cardiovascular benefits. Slower walking (at 2 miles per hour) was beneficial for older women, those with heart problems and women recuperating from illness. Even slow walking burns 60 to 80 calories per mile, helping to control your weight.

Even though we emphasize exercise in this chapter, remember the importance of other factors that might prolong your life, such as stopping smoking, watching your weight and controlling your blood pressure. Spurts of exercise may be more harmful than helpful if you don't keep in shape. Be consistent. Make walking a lifetime habit!

- *Does it help to carry hand weights or wear ankle weights when walking?*

  Weights may increase your caloric expenditure, but they may also throw you off balance. If you are comfortable with weights, they probably will do no harm.

- *Is there a way to test my aerobic fitness?*

  Yes. Here's a chart developed by Dr. Rippe and his associates at the University of Massachusetts and reported in the University of California, Berkeley, *Wellness Letter*, February, 1987:

  If you are 30 to 69 and want to evaluate your general aerobic fitness level, walk 1 mile as fast as you can and time yourself. Compare your results with the following chart.

Aerobic Fitness Rating	Time to walk one mile
Excellent	Less than 11 minutes: 40 seconds
Good	11:41–13:08
High average	13:09–14:36
Low average	14:37–16:04
Fair	16:05–17:31
Poor	More than 17:32

- *I love to ride a bicycle for exercise. Do you have any suggestions to prevent injury to my joints, especially my knees?*

  1. Set your seat with your knee slightly bent at the bottom of the stroke. If your seat is too low, you lose power. Putting it so high that you have to reach for the pedal puts undue stress on your knee.

  2. It's best to pedal in a low gear which gives you more action and less stress. A regular cadence of 70 to 80 revolutions per minute will give you aerobic exercise.

  3. One word of caution, not about your knees, but about your head. Most serious cycling injuries involve the head. Wear a helmet and ride defensively. Many drivers cannot see a bicycle.

  Cycling is healthy, inexpensive, aerobic, convenient and well suited to midlife. Enjoy it!

- *At 53 I am still working. We live in an apartment. Our neighborhood is such that I don't dare go walking, especially at night. What kind of exercise can I do indoors?*

Here are a few suggestions:

1. Jump rope. You can take a rope anywhere, even when traveling. You may be surprised how intensive this exercise can be. Begin with about a dozen skips and steadily increase each day. Most women learned this skill as a child. To avoid boredom, workout in front of the TV, using the half-hour news program each day as your exercise time. Earphones enable you to enjoy your own music, or skip to a television aerobics program.

2. Rebounding. Mini-trampolines are inexpensive and are easier on your feet and joints than jogging or running.

3. Stationary bicycle. Bicycling, whether stationary or otherwise, will save strain on aching feet. This type of exercise is less intensive because it is non-weight-bearing. But it can be aerobic if you tighten the resistance lever against which you pump. You can purchase a book or magazine rack for your stationary bike if you wish to make this your reading or studying time.

4. Stairs. If you have stairs, you can obtain sufficient exercise walking or jogging up and down them for 20 to 30 minutes, 3 or 4 times a week.

5. In-house jogging or walking. Set up a course in your apartment or home. Either walk or jog for 20 to 30 minutes at least 3 times a week. This can be done even in an apartment. You can even do this in a hotel room when you travel.

6. Mall walking. Many shopping malls are now opening their doors early in the morning for people who wish to walk their corridor shielded from inclement weather and the threat of mugging. In some places mall-walking clubs have been organized. You'll soon become familiar with distances and set your own course.

- *My favorite sport is golf. Yet I have been told golf is a poor exercise because it requires so little effort.*

Golf is not an aerobic exercise, but 18 holes require several miles of walking. No one can argue about the fun involved, the sociability or the fact you can enjoy walking as an exercise while playing golf. Avoid golf courses that require using a golf cart. Let others pursue whatever sport they will and you stay with golf.

- *Is tennis too strenuous for me since I am over 50?*

  Tennis is about as strenuous as you care to make it. A fun game of doubles among a compatible foursome is often more fun than strain and is not considered an aerobic sport. But it will give you the kind of exercise you can enjoy and look forward to, especially if you have a game time set up at regular intervals.

- *I must admit racquetball is very intense for me, but I enjoy it immensely. As a menopausal woman, is it too strenuous for my heart or my joints?*

  If you have been enjoying it with no ill effects, the best thing you can do is continue the sport. Each woman must seek out the particular sport or exercise she enjoys and tolerates best.

  Many women have deterred the creeping deformities of arthritis by sheer tenacity in this, their favorite sport. You may find racquetball leaves you stiff the next day, but the fun of the game is worth it and keeps you limber.

- *My grandchildren want me to go backpacking with them, and I would like to go. Is this sport too strenuous for me in my 50s?*

  This depends upon the shape you are in. Agree to go with them, but set the date far enough ahead to allow you to get in shape. If you have been taking regular walks at a rapid pace, and especially if you have been jogging, you should have little difficulty shaping up. You can also practice by walking up and down stairs on a regular basis.

  Check ahead of time to see how far and how steep the climb is and how heavy your pack will be. You may have to plan on frequent stops, but this is usually part of the fun and sociability of backpacking.

꙳　　꙳　　꙳

Any exercise is an effort, but you'll soon find the exhilarating "high" it produces is worth it.

- *My daughter has been urging me to join her dance aerobics class. After watching them the other day, I wonder if this is not too strenuous for me at age 48. I have been extremely active and walk for 5 and even up to 10 miles at a time.*

Only you can decide if it is too strenuous. After watching these women performing their dance aerobics, you would probably agree they undergo a rigorous program. It may be fun for some, but it is definitely a *workout* for most participants.

The advantage in joining a group is that it obligates you to attend and exercise on a regular basis. Don't feel you must keep up with women in their 20s and 30s. If you are limber enough to do it, there should be no problem if you gradually work into it. Another advantage to these classes is they nearly always include a warm-up and a cool-down, something few women allow themselves when exercising alone.

We urge you to check with your physician before undertaking any exercise program.

- *My husband hates exercise and is not very sympathetic about my exercising. I don't like to leave him while I exercise, but I feel I must get out and move around rather than sit and watch television all the time.*

He may feel a little guilty about not exercising and feels even more guilty when he sees you are following a good fitness program. Don't be intimidated by his inactivity and do not give up your exercise program.

You may be able to entice him to walk with you. But do not insist or he may resist more vigorously than he does now. Try to describe to him the "high" that follows your exercise sessions.

- *Recently I have noticed jogging makes me cough. I have been a 2-pack smoker for 30 years. I know I should quit, but I never get beyond the verbal stage.*

Your coughing could definitely signal the beginning of serious trouble. We strongly urge you to quit, even if it means you must obtain help from your doctor. Because a cough is sometimes the first sign of irritation, you should also check with your physician without delay for the possibility of lung cancer. Quit-smoking clinics are helpful.

- *How good is a program of calisthenics for exercise? It seems most of the emphasis nowadays is on sports, walking, jogging or running. What has happened to the old-fashioned calisthenics?*

Aerobics with all of its variations, such as dance aerobics, swim aerobics, water aerobics, etc., is simply a form of calisthenics put to music. There's nothing wrong or old-fashioned about calisthenics. If you enjoy calisthenics, you should certainly continue with them on a daily basis, if possible. Calisthenics have the advantage of convenience. You do not depend upon others, and you do not require a gym. You can do them at home.

You may also find an exercise-along TV program on calisthenics. Or you can purchase tapes that will give you a regular workout to follow.

- *Is it better to run uphill or down?*

Believe it or not, it is easier on your joints to run uphill. As you go down a hill, you speed up, your stride lengthens and your foot strikes the ground with greater impact. It is easier for you to lose control and fall when you are running downhill.

Studies have shown when you jog on level ground, your foot strikes the ground with a force equal to at least 3 times your body weight. This force on your feet can easily double when you are jogging downhill.

In order to slow down, you must tense your muscles. This can give you muscle soreness or even "runner's knee," which is soreness behind your kneecap. You may find it better to zig-zag as you jog downhill to decrease the effects of the slope and lessen the strain on your body.

- *Any suggestions for walkers?*

Because most midlifers seem to settle into walking as their most preferred type of exercise, here are a few "Pointers for Walkers" as suggested in the University of California, Berkeley, *Wellness Letter*, February, 1987:

1. If you're inactive but healthy, start with mile-long walks at a pace of 3 miles per hour, 5 times a week. Over the course of a month, boost your distance to 3 miles at a pace of 4 miles per hour, 5 times a week.

If you can find a particular sport or exercise you enjoy, you'll anxiously look forward to it.

2. You can increase the aerobic benefits of brisk walking in two ways. Swing your arms so your upper body gets a workout. As you get used to walking, carry a 6-pound backpack or hand weights. You can substitute a briefcase or shopping bag for the backpack.

3. Don't ride when you can walk. Incorporate walking into your daily routine. If you must take public transportation, get off a few stops early and walk to your destination.

4. If it's too hot or cold outdoors, walk in your local mall or in any other climate-controlled environment. Many malls now have walking programs sponsored by the American Heart Association.

5. Put variety into your walking program. Take a companion along. Try a different route, particularly leading to hilly territory, which will boost the aerobic benefits. If you get tired, alternate fast walking with strolling. If you walk alone you should have a dog for protection.

6. You don't need special footwear, but don't walk long distances in soft, shapeless shoes. Walking shoes should have a shank (a rigid arch) as well as some cushioning for the heel and the ball of your foot. Shoes especially designed for walking can make walking more enjoyable. And, they may give your feet better support and better grip so there's less tendency to slip or fall on uneven terrain. Cotton socks will add to your comfort and absorb perspiration as well.

- *Is there any exercise that will help to overcome my low backache?*

  In older women, the low backache is due to bony changes in the vertebrae, bony protuberances, etc., that limit motion and make motion uncomfortable. There isn't much in the way of exercise that will relieve discomfort of this kind.

  However, many backaches are due to muscle spasm or muscle weakness. Exercises designed to strengthen back muscles will often help relieve this type of pain. Because your abdominal muscles also help support your body, exercises that strengthen your abdominal muscles will also help support your back and indirectly relieve backache.

ε&   ε&   ε&

Choose an aerobic exercise, one that pushes your heart beat to 75 percent of your maximum for 20 to 30 minutes, 3 or 4 times a week.

Any excess weight will also aggravate low backache, so you must be sure your weight is normal. Always use correct posture in standing, sitting and lifting.

If you are considering a rowing machine, don't!

Dr. Lynne Pirie (1986), Sports-Medicine Specialist at the North Phoenix Health Institute says, "Rowing machines are not recommended for women with low-back problems. Rowing places an extreme amount of pressure on the discs in the low back."

See your doctor for specific exercises for low-back pain.

- *Recently I've been told I am developing osteoporosis. Are there safe exercises I can do?*

To improve your bone mass—in addition to taking calcium and estrogen (see chapter on Osteoporosis, page 219)—exercise is very important. But the exercises may need to be modified as discussed in the following suggestions:

1. Safe exercises

    dancing—square and ballroom
    stationary bicycling
    swimming
    walking
    water exercising

2. Unsafe exercises

    jogging
    jumping
    rowing machine
    situps or other back-bending exercises
    skipping rope
    weight lifting

3. Posture is important

Avoid lifting, twisting or sudden forceful movements. Protect the lower back by using the legs to lift. Bend at the knees to reach low placed objects.

- *Because of my increased nervousness along with hot flashes, my husband has considered installing a hot tub for me to "soothe" my nerves. Is this a good idea?*

Saunas, steam baths and whirlpools are safe for relaxation if you use them prudently. But they are not for everyone. Definite limitations and precautions must be observed to avoid health risks.

Saunas are small, enclosed rooms designed to emit dry heat. Made of wood and containing heat-retaining stones, these rooms are heated to 170F to 190F and relative humidity is kept at 5 to 25 percent. Humidity varies according to how much water is poured upon the stones. Over 1-million saunas in Finland are used by 4-million Finns every day.

Steam baths feature moist air with a relative humidity of about 95 percent and a temperature of 120F.

Whirlpool baths are fill-and-drain tubs with no heating device. They feature a whirling current of heated water that shouldn't be above 100F but often is. Temperature is controlled by the amount of hot water added to the pool. Many oversized bathtubs in homes are equipped to deliver this current of heated water.

Hot tubs and spas are often made of wood or fiberglass. They usually have a heater with thermostatic controls to adjust the temperature.

Water has a greater ability to store and conduct heat than air. This is why a whirlpool feels hotter than a steam room or sauna.

Perhaps the greatest health risk for users of hot tubs and saunas occurs when people become overheated for too long. This can damage your heart muscle, your brain or your nervous system. There is special danger to those with high blood pressure and heart disease. An added hazard is the risk of fainting and hitting your head on a bench, floor or edge of the tub. You should definitely not exercise in a hot pool or sauna.

It's not advisable to enter a hot tub when you are already over-heated or dehydrated from intense exercise. Avoid food and alcohol just before or during use of the hot tub. Cool down first and save your Happy Hour for after your hot tub.

If you have heart disease, it's foolish to jump suddenly into a cold shower or snow immediately after leaving a hot tub. It is unwise for *anyone* because of the possibility of hidden heart trouble.

Skin infection is possible due to hot-tub exposure, especially if chlorine levels are not meticulously maintained and baths occasionally scrubbed. Benches of steam baths and saunas are potential sources of herpes-simplex infections. Avoid these by sitting on your own personal towel.

In short, hot tubs and saunas are not the best answer for hot flashes—try estrogen!

- *Are there any exercises that will help get rid of my bulging stomach? Ever since I had my children, I have had a "pot belly.*

Exercises will help. Keep in mind that muscles are not strengthened in a mere few days. You will have to work at it, slowly, gradually but always increasing the repetitions.

If you still have a "pot" after 6 months of conscientious exercising, you may want to talk to your doctor about a tummy tuck. When the skin has been overstretched or when there is a separation of your abdominal muscles, leaving a hernia between, surgery may be required to correct the defect. But don't consider plastic surgery until you have rid yourself of excess fat and exercised consistently for at least 6 months.

10

Fertility & Menopause

In general, when you have not had a menstrual period for a year, you can stop worrying about pregnancy and stop using birth control. Remember the reason you stop having menstrual periods at menopause is that you run out of eggs in your ovaries. Without an egg, it is impossible to hatch a chick.

It is true you might rarely have a "dying-gasp" ovulation, in which an egg is released from the ovary after you have already stopped having menstrual periods. But this is very unusual. This is why we recommend you use contraception for a year after your menstrual periods stop. One year should allow for any uncommon, unwelcome ovulatory gasps.

- *Do women become less fertile as they get older?*

Most women do. In general, women are less fertile at 35, for instance, than they were at 18 or 20. Likewise, you should be less fertile at 45 than 25, but don't take a chance!

Age and fertility have become more important as women have become career-oriented, deferring their childbearing until they are established in the business world. Some of these women are discovering to their dismay they cannot become pregnant at 35. It is possible they could have become pregnant at an earlier age.

- *I am 50 and still having very normal, regular menstrual periods. My health is excellent. I am not the worrying kind, but just for the record, can I still get pregnant?*

Yes, you can. Because you are nearing the end of the egg supply in your ovaries, it might be difficult to get pregnant at this late date. However, if you do not want to become pregnant, continue to use contraception until you have had no menstrual periods for a year. After that time you should be able to relax and stop worrying about the possibility of pregnancy.

- *I have had no menstrual periods for over a year, even though I am only 44. My mother also stopped menstruating at 43. How safe am I as far as getting pregnant is concerned?*

  Given your mother also went through menopause at 43, you can assume you have run out of eggs in your ovaries and should be safe from pregnancy. An FSH (follicle-stimulating hormone) blood test, if the level is elevated, would indicate you are menopausal and therefore beyond your fertile state.

- *I have used birth-control pills for 20 years and continue to use them. I am 42 and wonder if I will continue to have menstrual periods as long as I take birth-control pills.*

  As long as you take your birth-control pills you will have menstrual periods. The estrogen in the pill will cause the lining of the uterus to build up each cycle, then be shed as the menses. We advise women to use only low-dose birth-control pills after 40 if they are healthy and non-smokers. We recommend that smokers switch to another form of birth control.

- *I am now 50 and have not had a menstrual period for over 4 months. Although I have taken special precautions not to get pregnant, I worry. How can I be sure?*

  A pregnancy test is inexpensive and will relieve your mind. You may also want to have an FSH (follicle-stimulating hormone) blood test to tell whether you have stopped ovulating and are menopausal.

- *I've taken birth-control pills for 20 years. Now I am 45, I worry about whether they will cause me to remain fertile longer than normal. if I discontinue my birth-control pills at 52, would I get pregnant?*

  If you are average, you will run out of eggs by 50 or earlier. At this point you would no longer be fertile, regardless of whether you have taken birth-control pills or not.

  Healthy non-smoking women may continue low-dose birth-control pills until they are menopausal. If you wish to discontinue your birth-control pill, consult your doctor about alternative

ð¢   ð¢   ð¢

If you have not had a menstrual period for a year or more during your menopause, you can stop using contraception.

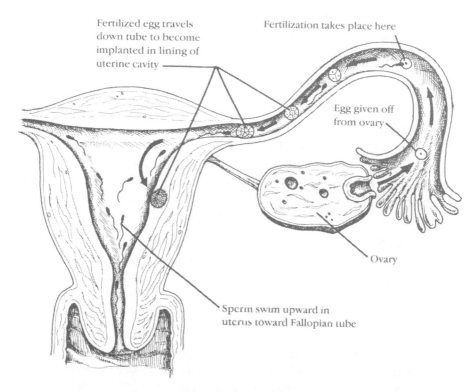

Fertilized egg travels down tube to become implanted in lining of uterine cavity

Fertilization takes place here

Egg given off from ovary

Ovary

Sperm swim upward in uterus toward Fallopian tube

Fertilization takes place in the fallopian tube. Then the fertilized egg makes its way down the tube to become implanted in the lining of the uterus. If it becomes trapped on the way, a tubal pregnancy may occur.

methods of birth control if your FSH is not elevated.[1]

- *Will birth-control pills increase my chance of developing cancer?*

  No. There is increasing evidence that birth-control pills decrease the risk of ovarian and endometrial cancers. Other benefits of birth-control pills include:[1]

1. Less anemia from menstrual blood loss.

2. Less irregular or heavy menstrual flow.

3. Reduced risk of benign breast disease (fibrocystic).

4. Reduced risk of uterine fibroids.

5. Reduced incidence of ovarian cysts.

---

1   Mischell, D.R. "Contraceptive Practices in Older Women." *Obstetrics and Gynecology Audio Digest.* October 5, 1990. Vol. 37, No. 19.

6. Less menstrual cramps.

7. Less risk of tubal pregnancies.

8. Less risk of tubal infections.

9. Decreased premenopausal bone loss.

- *Do you recommend I discontinue my birth-control pills and switch to a diaphragm, for instance, now I am 48? Otherwise how will I know when I am through menstruating and will not become pregnant?*

A diaphragm is a good way to get off the pill and get on with menopause. When your menstrual periods stop, you should continue to use contraception for another year. If you have no menstrual periods during that year, you can discontinue contraception forever.

- *I went through menopause at 49. I have had no menstrual periods since then until 3 months ago. About 4 months ago, at 53, I began taking estrogen and progestogen for osteoporosis and some hot flashes. I have resumed regular menstruation. Now I am wondering if I could get pregnant?*

The answer is a definite no! Your present menstrual periods represent "withdrawal" or artificial bleeding due to your estrogen-progestogen. This type of bleeding is common and normal. Although the bleeding may be inconvenient, you need not worry about pregnancy.

In general, when you decrease the dosage of estrogen to 0.625 milligrams per day (or the 0.05mg/day skin patch), you may find this is the smallest effective dose that will relieve your symptoms. This dose is also the smallest effective dose to prevent osteoporosis, so this may be a lifetime commitment.

When you are taking estrogen the amount of bleeding occurring each month normally will gradually decrease with time until it ceases altogether. In the meantime, you can be assured the lining shed from your uterus is not building up to bleed profusely at some future time or forming a cancer. The menstrual shedding (menstrual bleeding after menopause and during estrogen-pro-

≈ ≈ ≈

Women beyond 35 should switch from the pill to other methods of contraception, especially if they are smokers, diabetics or if they have high blood pressure.

gestogen replacement) is protective against cancer.

- *About a month ago I developed a clot in my leg and am still recovering from this episode. I have been taking the birth-control pill for many years. At 40, however, I definitely do not want to become pregnant. Yet my doctor insists I must stop taking birth-control pills because of the clot. Any suggestions?*

Birth-control pills increase the risk of clots. Because you have already developed one, you should discontinue taking the pills. There are other contraceptives, such as the diaphragm, condoms with creams, jellys or foam, the Norplant® System, as well as IUDs (intrauterine devices) such as the Progestasert® and the ParaGard®. Although the condom is less satisfactory for many males, it definitely makes sense in our present culture if you have sex with many partners.

You may want to consider tubal ligation. It is a procedure that can be performed with a laparoscope in the outpatient surgery of your local hospital. Your husband or partner could have a vasectomy. It is a mini-procedure that can be performed in a doctor's office under local anesthesia. Vasectomy entails far less risk than tubal ligation. That would make surgery for you unnecessary and might solve your problem.

- *I am 42 and have used the birth-control pill for many years. I have become aware I am in a high-risk category for serious side effects because of my heavy smoking. I have tried to quit smoking and failed miserably. What would you suggest?*

You are correct. We don't recommend birth-control pills for women of your age who are smokers, because of the threat of blood clots and myocardial infarction (heart attack). Talk to your doctor about one of the alternative methods of birth control.

Tubal ligation via laparoscopy is a simple outpatient procedure we recommend. Otherwise consider an IUD, Norplant® System (long-acting progestogen implanted in the inside of the upper arm), a diaphragm or a condom with jelly, cream or foam.

❧   ❧   ❧

Freedom from fear of pregnancy is one of the many "plusses" of menopause.

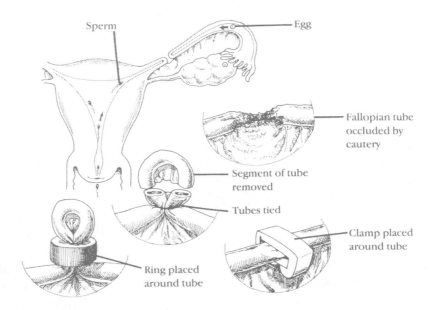

Sperm

Egg

Fallopian tube
occluded by
cautery

Segment of tube
removed

Tubes tied

Clamp placed
around tube

Ring placed
around tube

Some variations of sterilization by occluding (blocking) the fallopian tubes.

- *Ridiculous as it sounds, a friend of mine said she heard of a woman who conceived after a hysterectomy. Is this possible?*

  Perhaps anything is possible, but we have heard of only one such case. It's a medical oddity that the woman conceived just about the time of the hysterectomy and the embryo became implanted on the omentum (apron of fat) in the abdominal cavity. This one exception will be discussed (hopefully not anticipated) forever.

  After a hysterectomy there should be no channel through which the egg could meet the sperm and no nest (uterus) in which a fetus could rest or develop if conception did occur. Failures in tubal ligations (sterilization) are also rare.

- *You have spoken of running out of eggs at the time of menopause. If I have one ovary removed, am I only half as fertile?*

  No. One ovary functions just as well as two. Unless most of the second ovary is removed, you would still be just as fertile. When only a small part of an ovary is left there may be sufficient scarring so ovulation cannot take place and infertility results.

  If even a small part of your ovary is left, you will experience no evidence of menopause. That small part of ovary will secrete

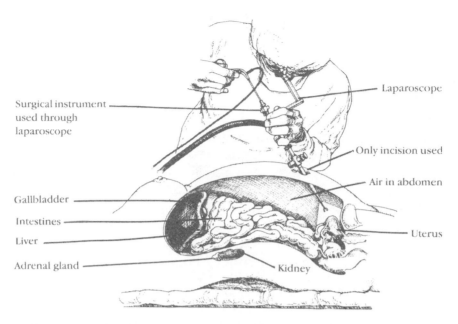

One-incision laparoscopy for exploration. Vision, light and instrument are all accommodated through the laparoscope, so only one incision is necessary.

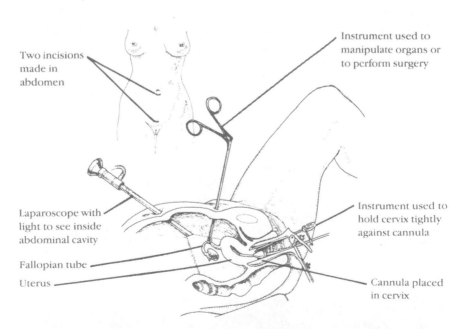

Two-incision laparoscopy as a method of sterilization.

sufficient estrogen (in most cases) to meet your needs. It takes very little hormone to prevent the unpleasant symptoms of the change of life.

- *What if I miss taking one of my birth-control pills? Will I accidentally get caught?*

Ordinarily one day's dose of birth-control pills can be missed without ovulation and consequent conception occurring. If you do miss taking one of your pills, take two the next day. If you miss two pills in a row, take two pills a day for several days. But you should also use additional contraception until your next menstrual period.

Be aware that you *can* conceive if you miss two days of mini-dose pills. If you are taking the mini-dose pills, you should try to take your pill at the same time (within 2 hours) each day.

- *If I have spotting between menstrual periods while taking the pill, should I switch to a different method of birth control?*

Instead of switching to a different method, you might switch to a different pill.

Some women require other than the usual dose found in birth-control pills. This is why there are so many different types and dosages. With the help of your doctor you can determine the right pill for you—one that will not cause you to have spotting between your menstrual periods.

- *I am 47 and still have regular menstrual periods. A friend of mine suggested I use an IUD (intrauterine device) for birth control until I am through menopause. Are IUD's safe?*

Progestasert® and ParaGard® IUDs are available. The Progestasert® must be replaced every year, but the ParaGard® only needs to be replaced every 6 years. The IUDs are best used by women with only one partner because of the increased risk of infection when there are multiple partners.

IUDs may provoke spotting and intermenstrual bleeding. This bleeding is especially distressing for women in midlife. Their

&a   &a   &a

In the past women usually bore the burden of providing contraception. The threat of sexually transmitted diseases in modern culture changes all of that because a condom offers the best protection.

estrogen level may already be waxing and waning, causing extra worry about the presence of cancer.

In addition to the high cost of IUDs, the devices come with a detailed consent form. It is important that women fully understand the risks involved in choosing this form of birth control.

- *I already have a Lippes Loop IUD. I am 48. Should I have the loop removed?*

In general, if you are having no problems, leave the IUD in place for a year after your menstrual periods stop. At that time you can have it removed and no longer have to worry about getting pregnant. Talk this over with your doctor because he may have a different approach to your question.

- *I am 45 and have just remarried. My 3 children are all married and have children of their own. My husband, who is 10 years younger than I, insists we have one child before I go through menopause. What about the risk to me as well as a baby born to someone my age?*

You may find you cannot conceive at your age. Fertility definitely decreases as you grow older. If you and your husband have mutually decided you want a baby, you should be aware of the increased incidence of Down's Syndrome: 1 in 32 at age 45. You should be prepared to have an amniocentesis during pregnancy and to face the decisions a positive result would entail.

The risks are definitely increased as you get older and especially at age 45. This is a growing problem, because so many women are waiting until they have established a career before having their family. It is estimated that over 200,000 over-35 women in the United States had their first baby in 1987.

A colleague of ours delivered a 50-year-old woman's first baby, a normal one. She conceived again (against her physician's advice) a few months later but had an abortion because of positive amniocentesis for Down's Syndrome. She conceived once more and delivered a normal infant. She consented to a tubal ligation at the time of this last delivery. We have wondered how long this superwoman might have continued to have babies!

11

Emotional Health & Menopause

As you near the menopause and estrogen levels decline, you may begin experiencing some subtle changes in the way you feel emotionally. These feelings may be more pronounced as the estrogen deficiency progresses. Symptoms may include: decreased energy and drive, mood fluctuations, difficulty concentrating, insomnia, headaches, irritability, aggressiveness, sense of internal frustration, inadequacy, nervous exhaustion, intolerance to loneliness, antisocial-behavior patterns, tension, depression, introversion, anxiety and marital troubles.[1] [2]

Other factors that may influence how you respond are the many changes that may be occurring in your life that can be unsettling. If children have married and left home, you may feel empty and unneeded. By contrast, you may feel the stress of children who are too comfortable (financially and otherwise) at home and do not want to leave home and fend for themselves.

Your own parents may be reaching an age of declining health that makes ever-increasing demands on your time and attention. You may have to seek a job outside your home simply to avoid both parent-sitting and baby-sitting.

Your partner may also be faced with stress. He may either share or occasionally unload some of this stress on you.

It is common to notice some memory loss as you become older. But this problem does not necessarily begin with menopause. If you observe carefully, you will notice it in your children who now may be in their 20s. Look around and you will also notice an occasional memory lapse in others your age and older.

1 Utian, W.H. "Biosynthesis and Physiologic Effects of Estrogen and Pathophysiologic Effects of Estrogen Deficiency: A Review." *American Journal of Obstetrics and Gynecology.* 1989. 161:128-31.
2 Dennerstein, L. "Psychologic Changes." *Menopause.* Yearbook Medical Publishers. 1987. 115-126.

Unless memory loss becomes alarmingly severe and embarrassing, you are most likely about average and normal. Paying a little more attention to details and conversation might help you to be less forgetful. Write down a schedule to follow each day and leave reminders where you need them. This is not a sign of senility—it is a sign of an organized person.

One of the authors, Dr. Mary Beard, changed specialties from Internal Medicine to Obstetrics and Gynecology at age 41. She found it necessary to rediscipline her mind and memory as she returned to residency training. Remember the advantage of experience and maturity you have over younger women.

- *I am having a bad time accepting wrinkles and, I suppose, aging altogether. Any suggestions?*

You will probably find acceptance by others follows acceptance by yourself. If you truly find wrinkles are giving you that much trouble, you may want to look at Chapter 14. Much can be done by way of plastic and cosmetic surgery to help.

But before you undertake surgery, go to the beauty parlor and ask them for a new hair-do. Then get a friend or even a cosmetologist to give you a new look to go with the hair-do. When they are through with you, you may find more radical methods are not necessary.

- *At 52 I find myself crying for no reason at all. My embarrassment at crying just makes me cry more. I have blamed it on menopause, but now I am worrying about my sanity.*

Fragile feelings are often a sign of stress, fatigue or depression. If this crying is accompanied by hot flashes, nervousness and insomnia, you have a right to associate it with menopause. Reliable studies have indicated hot flashes during sleep interfere with REM sleep (rapid eye movement sleep or deep, restful sleep). This can result in sleep deprivation which causes fatigue. Fatigue may cause more flashes and irritability. Thus the cycle feeds on itself.

Are you getting enough rest? Are you under pressure in your job or at home? Are you worried about your children, even though

ᕒ   ᕒ   ᕒ

Gradual memory loss may be a normal part of aging—it is not necessarily due to menopause.

they are married and out of your home by now? Are you worried about elderly parents who are becoming more of a responsibility for you? Are you taking estrogen or any other medication? If you aren't taking estrogen, perhaps you should be.

- *I seem so depressed lately. Is depression a normal part of menopause?*

It can be. Aging and estrogen deficiency are related to alterations in the brain chemicals (catecholamine and serotonin). Low levels of these chemicals have been shown to be associated with depression. Sleep deprivation because of hot flashes can also result in depressive symptoms.

Any treatment that raises the level of these chemicals prevents or relieves depression.

Exercise helps increase these chemicals (catecholamines and beta-endorphins).[3] Estrogen also increases the levels of these chemicals and stops hot flashes so the normal REM sleep pattern can be restored. There are medications available for depression.

Because we have excellent medications to relieve symptoms of depression, it seems a pity to continue without help.

- *I just had my 48th birthday. Everyone commented on how healthy I look. They don't know I spend hours most nights, worrying about a nervous breakdown or losing complete control over my emotions. Usually I wake up in a cold sweat. What is wrong?*

The most important thing about you and your condition is you know something is wrong. If you were not aware you were having difficulty, you would be in serious trouble. You are in contact with reality and want to do something about your anxiety.

It is not abnormal to be stressed or anxious when there is a reason for it. Don't be afraid to tell your husband about this or to discuss it with your best friend. But then you should seek help from your physician, who will either treat you herself or refer you to some-

&. &. &.

Depression is common during an "untreated" menopause (without ERT). But it could also be caused by one of several other conditions, such as diabetes.

3 Shangold, M.M. "Exercise in Menopausal Women." *Obstetrics and Gynecology.* 1990. 75:53S.

one else for treatment.

There are so many new medications which provide excellent relief from these emotional symptoms, it is foolhardy and unnecessary to suffer from them.

- *I have always been full of self-confidence and optimism. Lately I find myself slipping into negativism and despondency. It is almost as if I were a different person from my normal self. At 47 I wonder if I am losing my mind. Do other women of my age experience these feelings?*

You are not alone. Many women notice such changes during menopause. The important thing is to realize you are *not* losing your mind. It sounds more like you are becoming depressed. Depression, if it is caused by lack of estrogen, responds to estrogen-replacement treatment.

Even if your depression is not due to lack of estrogen, keep in mind we have some marvelous new medicines that can relieve depression. Check with your doctor who can determine if it is estrogen deprivation or if you need other medicines. You *can* be helped!

- *Ordinarily I can cope with most emergencies, and we have had our share. Recently my husband lost his job at 50, and it has thrown me into a tailspin. I am 48—is my reaction due to the menopause?*

Sometimes women are more fragile during this period of life—both physically and emotionally. One of our patients at age 49 suddenly had a married son and his 4 children move in with her and her husband. She couldn't turn them out. She couldn't cope with the burden of children and confusion at her age. She felt boxed in.

Her irritability and nervousness escalated into panic attacks, for which she took tranquilizers (her neighbor's). She withdrew from family and all social contacts. She secreted herself in her bedroom and wept frequently.

After 1-1/2 years of this, her son finally moved out along with his family. We stopped all tranquilizers and began to give her estrogen by way of transdermal patches.

Slowly this woman has recovered her equilibrium, come out of her room and begun to socialize. She and her husband are now making plans for an extended trip.

Sometimes women can stand menopause without stress, or they

can cope with stress without menopause. But when the two press upon them at the same time, it often proves to be more than they can stand.

If situations develop that threaten your health, if pressure is more than you can endure, you and your husband should find some alternatives that will permit you to function and not succumb— before things get completely out of control.

If you have skills, perhaps you can find a job. If not, you may want to train and prepare for a job. The fact you (and your husband) are doing something about your situation will help stop your "tailspin" and help you cope with your situation.

• *Recently I read an article on Alzheimer's disease. Some of the symptoms seem to fit me at 56. Is Alzheimer's disease an emotional condition?*

No. Alzheimer's disease is characterized by some definite organic changes in the brain. The main difficulty is this disease can only be accurately diagnosed at autopsy. Here are a few of the changes which are found:

1. Neurofibrillary fibers in the brain cells are tangled, just like a mussed head of hair.

2. There are plaques of degenerated nerve material.

3. Nerve cells become filled with vacuoles (cavities) that contain fluid and granular material.

All three of these processes are signs of degeneration and wasting. As this destructive process spreads, mental function decreases. As the chemical changes increase, the brain shrinks. Intellectual functioning and memory are disturbed.

• *How would I know if I were developing Alzheimer's disease?*

Unfortunately, symptoms vary widely from patient to patient and from day to day in the same person. Loss of memory seems to be a universal symptom. Terribly frustrating to both the patient and to those around her is the unpredictability of symptoms.

Early in the disease, it is not uncommon for an Alzheimer patient to exhibit garbled, almost nonsensical speech and complete loss of memory one day. Yet she may be completely lucid and able to carry on an intelligent conversation the next.

ᐧ᷂   ᐧ᷂   ᐧ᷂

Gradual memory loss is a normal part of aging.

Think how disturbing it would be to have forgotten how much you loved someone or how much joy you had with them or be completely unable to recognize those closest to you. Worse still, how would it feel to behave in an unpredictable, uncontrollable, socially unacceptable manner? We must be charitable and understanding to those affected by this disease.

- *What is the usual course of Alzheimer's disease?*

There are four phases; each individual may be affected differently.

1. At first, family and friends may not perceive anything serious is wrong. All they notice is easy fatigue, less energy and drive and a tendency to withdraw from strangers and from demanding situations. The victim may be aware something is wrong but doesn't know what. Frustration may produce anger over minor things, perhaps to hide embarrassment over memory loss.

2. In the second phase, slowed speech may be noticed. She may misunderstand what is said, miss the point of the conversation or the thread of a story. It's common not to be able to balance the check book, yet hesitant to admit it.

3. In the third phase, she becomes disoriented easily, forgetting both time and events. She may have had a delightful time at a party, yet forget she had ever been there. She may accurately recall the past, but is unable to recognize those around her.

4. In the fourth phase, the patient fails to recognize even those very close to her, such as her spouse and children. It is not uncommon in this phase for her to be unable to find her way around a house she has lived in for many years.

Deterioration of the brain may have proceeded so far she cannot even feed herself. From here on, it gets worse: Incontinence, depression, delusions and even delirium may follow.

Except for the early stages, the victim often does not know what is happening to her and, therefore, probably will not know it is Alzheimer's. From a medical standpoint, we still don't have good methods to diagnose Alzheimer's other than by autopsy. It becomes a diagnosis by exclusion, especially from depression.

Patients with depression usually respond well to antidepressant drugs; Alzheimer's victims show no change. Depressed women worry about their depression, whereas Alzheimer's patients seem unaware anything is wrong. They will not admit their memory is bad or they have any intellectual loss, which they often have.

In conclusion, let us say menopause, as far as we know, does not cause or even increase the incidence of Alzheimer's disease. Alzheimer's may come with menopause, but only coincidentally.

We have excellent treatment for menopausal symptoms, but as yet we have no treatment for Alzheimer's disease.

- *I have heard diabetics are more likely to develop depression. Is this true?*

Yes. Perhaps it is discouragement that comes with the physical deterioration caused by diabetes or the actual deterioration itself. At any rate, depression is often an unrecognized side effect of diabetes and has nothing to do with menopause.

- *I have been taking a mild tranquilizer that seems to control my postmenopausal emotional symptoms fairly well. If I am doing all right on this treatment, why should I start ERT?*

Discomfort from menopausal symptoms is no longer the *primary* reason for taking ERT (estrogen-replacement therapy). The most important reasons for taking ERT are to protect you against osteoporosis and cardiovascular disease.

ERT will also prevent the dryness, cracking and general atrophy of your vaginal tissues that usually occur when your body no longer produces estrogen.

12

Estrogen & Menopause

Estrogen first appeared for medical use in the 30s and was used by only a few doctors by the 40s. It was well into the 50s and 60s before estrogen really caught on and its tremendous value in treating menopausal symptoms was appreciated. At last menopausal women were offered relief from their distressing nervousness, hot flashes and insomnia!

Then in 1975 several researchers (Smith, Ross, Donovan, Herrman, Ziel and Finkle) published articles in the New England Journal of Medicine that confirmed estrogen's role in the development of cancer of the lining (endometrium) of the uterus. Earlier statistics and studies had missed this link because they had used only women whose uteri had been removed.

Because both doctors and patients were hesitant to give up this godsend to menopausal women, the risk was debated vigorously in various medical symposia. Ultimately these findings were verified. Everyone had to admit estrogen *did* increase the incidence of cancer of the endometrium.

When the Food and Drug Administration insisted warning inserts accompany all prescriptions for estrogen, women began to panic, worrying whether they had done irreparable harm to their bodies by taking estrogen. No doctor wanted the risk of prescribing estrogen, regardless of the severity of menopausal symptoms. Once more women were told to "tough it out," or they were given tranquilizers if they insisted on relief.

Diagnostic D&Cs (scraping of the lining of the uterus) were carried out on countless women to reassure them and their doctors they did not have endometrial cancer. Indignation mounted in women to think their trusted physicians would prescribe a hazardous cancer-producing drug for them.

When the FDA findings were finally published, it was shown that endometrial cancer risk was about 4 to 8 times greater in estrogen users. What too many physicians and patients *failed to consider* was the fact that endometrial cancer is relatively uncommon, treatable and causes very few deaths. In addition, endometrial cancers caused by estrogen are considerably more treatable and curable than spontaneously occurring endometrial cancers.

The increased incidence of endometrial cancer was still only 3 per 1,000, and the 5-year cure rate was more than 95 percent. Because endometrial cancer is likely to produce abnormal uterine bleeding early in its course, this type of cancer is one of the more successfully treated cancers because of early diagnosis.

Your risk of dying from cancer of the endometrium due to the use of estrogen is less than 0.23 per 1,000 women per year or less than 1 in every 4,300 women exposed. The silver lining to this dark cloud for menopausal women appeared with the discovery that if another hormone is added for 12 to 13 days during each month of estrogen, there is practically *no* increase in the incidence of endometrial cancer. This hormone is synthetic progesterone (also called *progestogen* or *progestin*) medroxyprogesterone acetate (Provera®) 10mg, norethindrome acetate (Norlutate®) 5mg or Micronor®.

Physicians now know that osteoporosis (thinning, brittleness of bone) with its severe fractures is a threat far worse than endometrial cancer. Osteoporosis affects at least 1 in 3 or perhaps even 1 in 2 of the 40-million postmenopausal women in the United States. Osteoporosis is responsible for at least 1.3- to 1.7-million fractures each year, including most of the approximately 250,000 hip fractures that occur in people over age 65. About one-quarter of those who break their hips die of complications within six months and another one-third enter long-term care and never regain social or physical functioning. Perhaps because of greater bone mass, black women are at much less risk of developing osteoporosis.

Another consideration is that cardiovascular disease is the leading cause of death in women—surpassing the rates of cancer and other diseases. Estrogen protects against the development of cardiovascular disease by lowering cholesterol: decreasing LDL

&&   &&   &&

Depression is common during "untreated" menopause without the benefit of estrogen-replacement therapy. It could also be caused by one of several other conditions, such as diabetes. Depression is one of the seldom-mentioned side effects of diabetes.

cholesterol, raising HDL cholesterol and having direct effect on the blood-vessel walls. There is a 50% or greater reduction in cardiovascular disease and related deaths for women on ERT.[1]

Researchers disagree on the possible added risk of breast cancer linked with longterm estrogen use. Recent reviews suggest that any increased breast-cancer use due to estrogen use is small, if it exists at all.[2]

Estrogen has been indicted, put on trial and now vindicated. Or we might say it has been paroled into the custody of the progestogens. The two hormones should be prescribed together in a cyclic fashion or taken daily continuously by any woman who has her uterus..

- *If my menopausal symptoms are tolerable, is there any reason I should take estrogen?*

One of the foremost authorities on estrogen, Dr. Lila Nachtigall (1986), claims estrogen will actually prolong your life because it decreases the likelihood of strokes and heart attacks. It also slows down the progression of osteoporosis, with its high rate of fractures, deformities (humping of the back) and deaths due to complications of these fractures.

With few exceptions, estrogen is beneficial to all women after menopause, regardless of their symptoms.

- *If I take estrogen, will it prolong my menopause? Am I merely deferring the inevitable by taking it? Won't I have to go through menopause sometime?*

Estrogen or ERT will not prolong or defer menopause. Your ovaries will "run out" of eggs as usual. You will go through menopause, but you will not have its unpleasant symptoms.

Yes, you may continue to have menstrual periods for a while, but this "withdrawal" bleeding is lighter than normal periods and stops eventually. An FSH (follicle-stimulating hormone) blood level can tell us when you have actually completed menopause.

1 Lobo, R.A. "Cardiovascular Implications of Estrogen Replacement Therapy." *Obstetrics and Gynecology.* 1990. 75:18S-25S.
2 Lufkin, E.G., et al. "Estrogen Replacement Therapy: Current Recommendations." *Mayo Clinic Proceedings.* 1988:27:201-23.

- *Is estrogen vaginal cream considered as ERT? In other words, can I assume vaginal cream can take the place of estrogen by mouth or skin patch?*

  Vaginal cream is a form of ERT, but it is absorbed unevenly. Therefore it is inadequate as far as supplying enough estrogen to prevent osteoporosis and cardiovascular disease. Except where there is only a small loss of estrogen, vaginal cream will not relieve vasomotor symptoms (hot flashes, nervousness and insomnia). Ordinarily, if you require vaginal cream, you also need a greater dose of estrogen by some other route to meet these additional demands for estrogen in your body.

- *I am 54 and have had repeated urinary infections for the last 2 or 3 years. Is it likely estrogen might help prevent these infections?*

  Yes. Of course you should have your doctor check to see which organisms are causing the infections. If they appear to come without a positive culture, they may be due to changes in the vaginal and urinary tissues. Such irritations will readily respond to estrogen. Check with your doctor to see if estrogen deficiency could be the cause of your problem. You should be taking ERT anyway to prevent osteoporosis and decrease your chances of heart attack and stroke.

  Women who have frequent urinary infections before menopause may require a FSH (follicle-stimulating hormone) blood test to see if estrogen deficiency is a contributing cause of their irritation. Don't forget to have your sex partner checked for infection; he could be causing your repeated urinary infections.

  Be sure you drink plenty of water, preferably 2 quarts a day. Concentrated urine is more likely to become infected.

  After emptying your bowels, wipe from front to back to avoid carrying bacteria from your rectum to your vagina and urethra.

  Cranberry juice helps in certain cases. Because cranberry juice is excreted as an acid into the urinary tract and because acid urine is less likely to become infected, drink cranberry juice to help clear up bladder irritations and infections. Cranberry juice is less expensive than medicine, but medication may also be necessary.

  And while we are on this cranberry kick, let us mention yogurt is also beneficial. It contains lactobacilli which encourage the growth of friendly bacteria in the vagina and colon. You may also want to talk with your doctor about taking a medication—such as Macrodantin®—to prevent infections after intercourse.

- *I am 56 and have never taken estrogen. I have had no problems in my vagina, such as drying, itching or tenderness with sex. Why do I need ERT?*

It may take up to 15 years for these changes to appear, but nearly every woman will experience them eventually. You should take ERT not only to deal with these changes, but also to prevent osteoporosis and lessen your chances of developing cardiovascular disease (heart attacks and strokes).

- *Does vitamin E help hot flashes?*

There are those who claim it does. Subjective symptoms and their relief are often difficult to identify, evaluate or prove. Vitamin E in the recommended dosages will do you no harm.

- *I am 59, feel wonderful and have no menopause symptoms, such as hot flashes, insomnia or nervousness. Surely you don't think I should take estrogen. I was brought up believing "If it works, don't fix it!"*

Although you feel well, there are some changes going on in your body that do need "fixing" or at least they need to be stopped. A growing amount of information suggests a protective effect upon your system by estrogen in two significant areas: your heart and your bones.

It is an established fact women before menopause have fewer heart attacks than men. After menopause—without the protective effect of estrogen—women are just as prone to heart attacks as men. Recent studies indicate ERT (estrogen-replacement therapy) can help maintain this premenopausal low rate of heart attacks.

In addition to the beneficial effects of estrogen upon your cardiovascular system, estrogen can put a "hold" on osteoporosis. Thus it prevents hip and wrist fractures as well as humping of your back due to fractures of your vertebrae. ERT is no longer a matter of merely relieving nuisance complaints (nervousness and hot flashes) but a matter of life and death.

- *What about the increased pigmentation on my cheeks when I used birth-control pills. Will I get the same effect from ERT?*

Birth-control pills contain up to 10 times as much estrogen as ERT. The progestogen contained in the pills is often the culprit in causing pigmentation.

- *I read a magazine article that recommended women who take estrogen should do so for only a minimal length of time and use the minimal dose to relieve their symptoms. Do you agree?*

ERT is a lifetime commitment. Most research shows ERT gives lifetime protection against osteoporosis. It also helps you live longer, because it gives some protection against heart attacks.

As far as the dose is concerned, it has been found that 0.625mg of conjugated estrogen orally every day (or the 0.05mg/day skin patch) along with 12 to 13 days of progestogen—if you have a uterus—will give adequate protection against osteoporosis. It may be necessary to give larger amounts at first to relieve the vasomotor symptoms of menopause (hot flashes, nervousness, insomnia), especially when they are due to removal of the ovaries before the normal onset of menopause.

- *I am 80. My doctor put me on ERT a few months ago to combat vaginal irritation and tenderness with sex. He also said it would help put my osteoporosis on hold. The trouble is I have started to have menstrual periods again. Could I get pregnant? Will the periods continue as long as I take ERT?*

You will not be able to become pregnant. You used up all your eggs long ago when you first went through menopause. Your periods may continue for a few months, but they will gradually become lighter and lighter. For most women they will eventually stop altogether.

If your periods do not stop, then your doctor may want to give you 2.5mg of medroxyprogesterone daily with your 0.625mg of conjugated estrogen or your 0.05mg/day Estraderm® patch. The lining of your uterus should become atrophic (dry up) in 3 months (or in 9 months at most) and your menstrual periods will stop.

- *I am 52. My doctor started me on estrogen a few months ago to relieve some of my hot flashes. But he said nothing about progesterone. Should I be taking it?*

You didn't say whether you still had your uterus. No woman who still has her uterus should take estrogen without also taking progestogen. Otherwise she might develop endometrial hyperplasia (thickening of the lining of the uterus) which could turn into cancer. If you don't have a uterus, progestogens are probably not needed. There is concern that progestogens may decrease the beneficial effects of the estrogens on the cardiovascular system.[3]

- *Why do doctors recommend stopping estrogen for a few days each month?*

One of the several methods of prescribing estrogen has been to give it 25 days each month along with a progestogen from the 16th to the 25th day of the month. Both were stopped after the 25th day to allow withdrawal bleeding. Some women tolerate this well, but others develop symptoms when they are not taking estrogen. Taking estrogen daily without stopping and then adding the progestogen from the 1st to the 12th of the month is just as effective, easier to remember and eliminates the symptoms seen from the 25th to the end of the month. The withdrawal bleeding will occur after the completion of the progestogen in the middle of the month.

- *Is there any significance to clots in menstrual flow?*

Ordinarily nature provides sufficient anticoagulant in the menstrual blood to keep your menstrual flow from clotting so it can pass easily through the cervix and into the vagina. If clots appear, it usually means excessive bleeding (more than the anticoagulant can handle) and may mean the bleeding should be investigated.

When taking ERT, any bleeding longer than 5 days, heavy bleeding or clots indicate a need for investigation by your doctor.

- *I phoned my doctor to complain about hot flashes, etc. He phoned in a prescription for estrogen. I am worried about cancer. What do you suggest?*

Before you are given estrogen, you should:

1. Have a thorough physical examination that includes a pelvic exam and a breast exam.

2. Have a Pap smear.

3. Have either a progestogen-challenge test or an endometrial biopsy to rule out hyperplasia or endometrial cancer.

4. Have a mammogram.

5. Have a urinalysis and hemoglobin or hematocrit tests.

6. Have a battery of blood tests that include blood sugar, liver function, thyroid function, triglyceride and cholesterol tests,

---

3 Lobo, R.A. "Cardiovascular Implications of Estrogen Replacement Therapy." *Obstetrics and Gynecology.* 1990. 75:18S-25S.

calcium and phosphorus levels.

7. Your family history is important to determine if you are at special risk of cancer or osteoporosis or cardiovascular disease.

- *I was taking estrogen with excellent relief of my menopausal symptoms. Recently my doctor added progestogen, because he said recent research showed a woman with a uterus should not take estrogen without progestogen. The problem is the progestogen gives me the same symptoms of PMS (premenstrual syndrome) I had before menopause. What should I do?*

Usually if you persist, the irritability and depression will pass away. If these symptoms continue to such an extent you cannot tolerate them, the dose of progestogen may have to be reduced. If the symptoms still persist, your doctor can try a different kind of progestogen.

Your doctor is correct. You should not take estrogen without taking progestogen.

- *Is it necessary to stop ERT occasionally just to give the pelvic organs a rest?*

No. Estrogen-replacement therapy is a lifetime commitment with many rewards for taking it. When it is discontinued, osteoporosis will progress and the risk of heart and cardiovascular complications resumes.

- *What happens if I skip a day's dose of estrogen or progestogen?*

Usually nothing. You can ignore it and simply get on with the next day's dose. It is not necessary, as with birth-control pills, to take twice the dosage the next day. The same thing would apply if you accidentally took your medicine twice in a day—ignore it.

If you have trouble remembering to take your hormone tablets, you may want to consider taking the estrogen in transdermal (skin patch) form.

- *What are the advantages of the skin-patch method of taking estrogen?*

1. The dose is taken in a controlled release rather than spasmodically as it would be when taken orally or as a shot.

2. It is easier to remember and more convenient.

3. This method of administration avoids a first pass through the liver. This reduces the risks of clotting, elevating the blood pressure and aggravating a damaged liver.

ESTROGENS, ORAL (Tablets), +	
Trade Name	*Dosages, milligrams (mg)*
Estrace	1mg, 2mg
Estratab, Menest	0.3, 0.625, 1.25, 2.5mg
Ogen	1mg, 2mg
Premarin	0.3, 0.625, 0.9, 1.25, 2.5mg

ESTROGEN, TRANSDERMAL (Skin Patch)	
Trade Name	*Dosages, milligrams (mg)*
Estraderm	0.05, 0.1mg/day

ESTROGEN, VAGINAL CREAMS	
Trade Name	*Dosages, milligrams (mg)*
Ortho-Dinestrol	1.5mg/gm
Ogen Cream	0.01% in 90gm
Premarin	0.625mg/gm

PROGESTOGENS	
Trade Name	Dosage, milligrams (mg)
Provera, Curretabs, Amen	2.5, 5, 10mg
Megace	20, 40mg
Norlutin, Nor-QD, Micronor	0.35, 5mg
Norlutate, Aygestin	0.35, 5mg
Ovrette	0.075mg

4. The skin patch avoids adverse reactions for those whose stomach does not tolerate oral estrogen.

5. An occasional skin reaction occurs in about 10 percent of women.

- *I read that women should not take birth-control pills beyond 35. I am still taking them at 45. In fact, I wouldn't think of giving them up for fear of getting pregnant. How dangerous are they?*

Healthy non-smoking women may continue low-dose birth-control pills until they are menopausal.[4] If you are a smoker, consider an alternative method of birth control such as the IUD, condoms, diaphragm, Norplant® System (long-term progestogen implants in the upper arm) or a tubal ligation.

4 Mischell, D.R. "Oral Contraception 1990: Taking Stock." *Dialogues in Contraception.* 1990.Vol. III, No. 1. 1-3.

- *What are the normal side effects of ERT?*

  In general estrogens are tolerated well by most women. Many of the symptoms disappear after one or two months. But those that persist need attention by changing the dose or the route of delivery (tablet to patch or vice versa).

  1. Withdrawal bleeding. When estrogen is given with 12-13 days of progestogen, 80%-90% of women[5] will have regular bleeding (menses) each month. The flow should be light and no longer than 4-6 days. Heavier flow or longer duration may require adjusting the estrogen or progestogen dose. If both estrogen and progestogen are given daily, fewer women experience monthly bleeding. Expect spotting for the first 3 to 9 months as the uterus lining becomes atrophic (dries up).

  2. Fluid retention. It is uncomfortable to be swollen and many women are distressed by weight gain. This symptom usually subsides if treatment is continued. Drinking 6 to 8 glasses of water each day, avoiding salt and walking 30 minutes each day may help to alleviate fluid retention. An occasional diuretic may be needed.

  3. Weight gain. Estrogens used for ERT are at the low end of what the menstrual cycle produces, so if you are exercising regularly and following a lowfat diet, weight gain should not be a problem.

  4. Breast enlargement and tenderness. In some women the increased size of the breasts will be welcome. But in others it becomes a problem as breasts become heavier and more uncomfortable. Often this enlargement is temporary, but it is a reason to give the smallest dose (0.625mg by mouth, or 0.05mg by skin patch.)

  Breast tenderness usually only lasts 1 to 2 months. If it persists, eliminate all caffeine, take 400 units of vitamin E daily and ibuprofen (600 milligrams) 4 times a day for a week or so. If it persists, talk with your doctor about changing the dose or the type of estrogen.

  5. Increased vaginal discharge. Just as too little estrogen produces dryness, increased estrogen in ERT may cause troublesome and annoying vaginal discharge. Only seldom is the discharge enough to require a small tampon or napkin.

5   Hammond, C.B. "Estrogen Replacement Therapy: What the Future Holds." *American Journal of Obstetrics and Gynecology.* 1989. 161:1864-8.

6. Headaches. These could be a manifestation of fluid retention throughout the entire body. It is usually temporary but may indicate too much estrogen. In this case the dose can be reduced. Some women who get headaches with the oral medications (tablets) have no headaches with the skin-patch application.

7. Nausea. Some women develop nausea due to estrogen. These are often the same women who have more nausea with pregnancy (perhaps because of the tremendous increase in the amount of estrogen in the blood during pregnancy). The nausea is seldom severe enough to discontinue treatment and seems to disappear with time.

If it persists, the dose, type of estrogen or the way the estrogen is taken (patch vs. oral) may need to be changed.

8. Sensitivity to estrogen. Occasionally a woman is so allergic to estrogen that she cannot take it at all. Unfortunately there is no good substitute for estrogen so far as genitourinary atrophy is concerned, but progestogen will stop hot flashes about 80% of the time. And, there is increasing evidence that progestogen may be effective in stopping the progression of osteoporosis.

9. Cramps. Some women experience cramps with the resumption of monthly withdrawal bleeding. Ibuprofen (600-800 milligrams) every 6-8 hours will relieve the cramps. If not, reducing the estrogen or progestogen dose may help.

10. Lower abdominal fullness or bloating. This symptom is usually seen the first couple of months after starting estrogen. Then it subsides. If it continues then the estrogen or progestogen dose may need to be reduced.

11. Irritability and aggressive behavior. This usually indicates the estrogen dose is too high. This may be seen as a problem with injectable estrogens, so using this form of estrogen is discouraged.

12. Nasal stuffiness. This does not occur often, but can be very irritating. Reducing the dose or changing the type of estrogen is often helpful.

           ⁋   ⁋   ⁋

Yes, you do feel better when you take estrogen!

- *Is it possible to become addicted to hormones? Can I become hooked on estrogen?*

The only withdrawal symptoms would be a recurrence of symptoms of menopause. Estrogens are not addicting in the sense narcotics are. But high doses of estrogen can give a woman euphoria (high sensation) and they become severely symptomatic (hot flashes, nervousness, agitation, insomnia, etc.) when the dosage is reduced to normal blood levels. Therefore, we discourage the use of injectable estrogens or any form of estrogen that gives extremely high blood levels.

- *Is there any reason I should avoid taking estrogen? Are there any side effects or hidden, little-known reasons I should not take estrogen?*

You should not take any medicine you do not need. But about 85 percent of women have unpleasant and troublesome symptoms of menopause severe enough to merit treatment. If you have had breast or endometrial cancer, active liver disease or recent blood clots in your legs, these are reasons not to take estrogen.

- *If only 10 percent of women have severe symptoms, why should the rest of us take estrogen?*

In the past, we avoided prescribing estrogen in women unless their symptoms were severe. But 85 percent of women have symptoms troublesome enough to require relief. In addition, the effects of osteoporosis and cardiovascular disease may be more serious than any ill effects from taking estrogen. There is a growing feeling that all women would benefit from taking estrogen to protect them from these devastating diseases. Osteoporosis caused 190,000 hip fractures in 1979 in the United States, 267,000 in 1980, and may cause over 500,000 fractured hips by the year 2000, along with a significant number of deaths due to complications (pneumonia, etc.) following these fractures.

Women who take estrogen—even for a short time—after menopause are 35% less likely to suffer hip fractures, according to a review of 2,873 women in the Framingham, Massachusetts Heart Study. And women taking it now are 66% less likely to suffer hip fractures in the next two years.

When you see older (and some who are not so old) women who suffer from a disfiguring humping of their backs and loss of height, you are seeing the result of fractured, crushed vertebrae due to osteoporosis. Add to this disfigurement the women who suffer from chronic backache for the same reason, and you begin to comprehend the ravages of osteoporosis.

At least 1 woman in 4 will have *severe* osteoporosis. Costs for treating these fractures and deformities in the United States run into billions of dollars each year. Gradually we have had to admit estrogen is *preventive* against osteoporosis and should be taken by most women. Add to this the protective effect of estrogen against heart attacks and stroke, and we have additional good reasons for taking estrogen. In women over age 65 33% die from heart disease, 17% from cancer and 1.5% from complications of hip fractures as a result of osteoporosis.[6] Death rates from coronary heart disease are four times those of endometrial and breast cancer combined.

- *I have had a hysterectomy along with removal of my ovaries. When I take estrogen I feel better. Is this reason enough to take estrogen?*

There are many reasons you should take estrogen.

1. You will feel better.

2. It will prevent all of the emotional, psychological and physical symptoms that accompany estrogen deprivation. See page 5.

When you review all of those symptoms, you will see convincing reasons why you should take estrogen.

- *Will estrogen cause me to gain weight? I know they give cattle estrogen to fatten them.*

Some women have a tendency to gain weight when they take estrogen. But many women without estrogen have a tendency to gain weight as they grow older. It will require both lowfat eating and exercise for many women to maintain their desired weight.

- *Will estrogen cause bloating and a feeling of fullness? My neighbor says this is one of her most unpleasant side effects of taking estrogen.*

Everyone reacts differently to different drugs, including estrogen. You may notice no unpleasant side effects, or you may have some you have never heard of. In general, the dose of estrogen can be adjusted to meet your needs without having any *serious* side effects bother you.

6   Utian, W.H. "Current Perspectives in Management of the Menopausal and Postmenopausal Patient: Introduction." *Obstetrics and Gynecology.* 1990. 75:1S.

If your doctor prescribes estrogen for you, keep in touch so he/she can regulate the dose to your special needs and tolerance.

- *Will estrogen cause breast cancer?*

Estrogen alone does not seem to be a carcinogen (cancer causer). There is some controversy as to the type of estrogen used (natural versus synthetic), the use of progestogen and other risk factors such as family history, smoking, high-fat diet, alcohol use, etc. that may increase the risk of developing breast cancer for those women using estrogen for longer than 15 years.

To quote one expert, "Estrogen has been vindicated as far as causing cancer of the breast.[7]

We do not give estrogen to women who have had breast cancer as it may stimulate growth of their breast cancer. You cannot relax your vigilance in checking your breasts each month and you need to have your yearly mammogram after age 50.

- *Will estrogen cause hair to grow on my face or make me appear more masculine?*

As you grow older and especially after menopause, testosterone (male sex hormone) may increase or at least express itself more in your body because of falling estrogen levels. One of the effects of testosterone is the growth of coarse hairs on your face. These coarse hairs are characteristic of menopause.

Instead of causing these hairs, estrogen may prevent their appearance. Remember estrogen is the "feminizing" hormone. It is the hormone that causes you to develop from a child into a young woman. It produces the rounding curves so typical of a woman, including the fullness of your breasts.

- *I would like to stop taking estrogen. But every time I decrease the amount or stop taking my pills entirely, I begin all over again with hot flashes and other menopausal symptoms. Is there any way to discontinue estrogen without all these problems?*

If you wish to discontinue taking estrogen, you must do so gradually. Check with your doctor. He may prescribe estrogen pills that are half or even one-fourth as strong. Decrease the dose

7   Nachtigall, L.E. "Estrogen Replacement Therapy and Breast Cancer." *Current Perspectives on Managing the Premenopausal and Postmenopausal Patient.* Dec. 1990. New York University Postgraduate Medical School Conference, Dallas, TX.

gradually each month until you are taking the smallest dose.

Next, you can take this smallest dose only every other day, then every third day, etc., until you discontinue the estrogen completely. Any symptoms you develop with such a program are usually minor.

Keep in mind some women continue to experience menopausal symptoms years after menopause each time they taper off or completely discontinue their estrogen. Before you discontinue your estrogen, check with your doctor. If you choose to discontinue estrogen, keep in mind the threat of osteoporosis and cardiovascular disease.

- *What about progestogen? How necessary is it to take this hormone along with my estrogen?*

It is necessary to protect the uterus as there is virtually no increase in endometrial cancer when estrogen is prescribed along with progestogen. Progestogen is taken for 12 to 13 days each month (Dr. Don Gambrell, 1983). This cyclic method of taking hormones makes sense because it simulates the normal processes of the menstrual cycle in your body.

- *What about estrogen applied to the body as a skin patch?*

Estrogen by patch is catching on. You apply a patch with the proper dose of estrogen to your abdomen—or some other area of your body if you prefer—twice a week. This method permits your body to absorb the estrogen at a steady rate and avoids taking pills every day. Sensitivity to the patch occurs in about 10 percent of women. Many women prefer this method over pill-taking.

As yet no patch has been developed for progestogen, because progestogen cannot be readily absorbed through the skin. But efforts are being made to develop such a compound for patch use. So, the progestogen your body needs must be taken in pill form.

- *Do tranquilizers work just as well as estrogen for relieving menopausal symptoms?*

In some cases they help, but it is the lack of estrogen that is producing the symptoms. Tranquilizers cause drowsiness and they can be addicting. In addition, tranquilizers may affect your driving alertness. They certainly should never be combined with alcohol in any amount. Tranquilizers certainly will not protect you against osteoporosis or cardiovascular disease.

- *My worst menopausal symptom is insomnia. I think I would prefer to take an occasional sleeping pill rather than start on estrogen.*

  Sleeping pills are addicting and what is now an occasional pill can easily become a habit. Usually the end result is an unwanted addiction to a pill along with a persistence of your insomnia. The decline or absence of estrogen causes the sleep disturbance by interfering with the normal REM (rapid eye movement that is typical of deep sleep) sleep pattern. Estrogen restores this sleep pattern if estrogen deprivation is the cause of the insomnia.

  When you can't sleep, get up and do something until you are sleepy. Otherwise you might try reading in bed until your eyes won't stay open.

  Don't stay in bed and roll and toss while you worry about not getting your rest. Avoid taking naps during the day or you will establish a pattern of sleeping during the day and tossing all night.

  Discuss your insomnia with your doctor. He may advise estrogen in place of sleeping pills. At least estrogen is not addicting.

- *Will estrogen improve my libido and my ability to achieve orgasm?*

  It may, but not necessarily. Some women find only a slight decrease, if any, in their libido during menopause. Many women experience an increase in both libido and orgasm because they no longer have to worry about pregnancy.

  For women with decreased libido and ability to orgasm, estrogen replacement is usually sufficient. It takes about 6 months and may require adjustment of the dosage and checking estradiol levels to be sure the estrogen levels are in a normal range. If there is still a problem after that time, a small dose of testosterone may be helpful.[8]

- *I have an excellent doctor, but she doesn't tell me much about the medicine she prescribes for me. As a result, I have many unanswered questions after I have had a prescription filled.*

  Here are a few questions you might ask (and you have a right to know) at the time your doctor gives you a prescription:

8   Beard, M.K.; Curtis, L.R. "Libido, Menopause and Estrogen Replacement Therapy." *Postgraduate Medicine.* 1989. 86:1:225-228.

1. Are there any side effects I should I look out for?

2. Will this conflict with any medicine I am already taking?

3. Are there any foods I should or should not take with this medicine?

4. Can or should this prescription be refilled?

5. Will this medicine conflict with my _____ (any condition you have besides the one for which the medicine is intended, such as diabetes, heart disease, etc.)?

6. When and how often should I take this medicine?

Knowing these facts, you can double-check the medicine you receive from the pharmacist and instructions on the bottle. Insist on getting the package insert. Mistakes are occasionally made.

- *I know individual needs vary, but what is the average amount of estrogen needed for relief of menopausal symptoms?*

In general, we give just enough estrogen to make you comfortable. Most women require 1.25 milligrams of conjugated estrogen, 0.1mg/day of the Estraderm® Patch. 0.2mg of Estrace®, or 1.25mg of Ogen® daily to relieve their symptoms. We may decrease this dose to 0.625 milligrams of conjugated estrogen daily (or the 0.05mg/day skin patch), 1mg Estrace® or 0.625mg Ogen® just to see if you can be kept comfortable on a smaller dose. If you have side effects from estrogen, such as a bloated feeling, we might try an even smaller dose.

- *What if I am unable to take estrogen at all? What if it makes me ill, nauseated or if I am allergic to it? Is there anything else that would relieve my hot flashes?*

Progestogen alone, the other hormone that is given for 12 to 13 days each month along with estrogen, relieves as much as 80 percent of the unpleasant symptoms (especially hot flashes). Belladonna may also relieve many of the vasomotor symptoms (hot flashes, nervousness, insomnia) of menopause.

Clonidine, a drug originally used to control high blood pressure, has also been shown to be about 50 to 60 percent as effective as estrogen in controlling the vasomotor symptoms of menopause. You may have more side effects with clonidine than with estrogen, but it is good to know we have one more alternative treatment to help you.

Minor tranquilizers will also give a certain amount of relief from the emotional symptoms of menopause. Wherever possible, we avoid these drugs because of possible dependency. For the same reason, we are careful to limit the number of pills you may have at one time.

You may find you can tolerate skin-patch estrogen when oral estrogen causes nausea.

- *What side effects can progestogens cause?*

Possible side effects include moodiness, cramping, nervousness, increased appetite, breast tenderness, headaches, depression, sudden onset of migraine headaches when stopping or starting the medication, and abdominal bloating.

Most women experience none or a few side effects. Observe how you feel for a couple of months. If symptoms persist, your doctor may change the dose, the kind of preparation or give a suppository. He/she may even prescribe a sublingual (under the tongue) tablet of natural progesterone instead of a progestogen tablet.

- *You have mentioned progestogen several times and the necessity of taking it along with estrogen. Can I also take progestogen as a skin patch?*

Progestogen is not yet available as a skin patch because progestogen is not well absorbed through the skin. Research on some promising new chemical processes may make progestogen become available in skin-patch form in the future.

- *What are the disadvantages of progestogen?*

Occasionally progestogen causes irritability, breast tenderness, fluid retention, increased appetite and moodiness. But these patients often overcome their discomfort if they persist in using the hormone. There are several brands of progestogen. When one brand does not agree with you, you may find another one does.

In general, the most commonly used brand is Provera®, taken as a 10-milligram tablet for 12 to 13 days each month. Your doctor may find you tolerate only 5 milligrams daily, in which case you will probably have to take it for 13 days a month. If you do not tolerate Provera in any dosage, your doctor may try you on

కæ   కæ   కæ

Estrogen increases libido in some women. For others it preserves the libido they have always had.

Norlutate® or some other brand of progestogen.

- *Are there times when I should take only progestogen?*

Yes. If you cannot take estrogen to relieve hot flashes, you may find progestogen alone will relieve most of them.

Progestogen is also a valuable medicine when taken as a "challenge test" when you are not having menstrual periods. You take it for 10 days to see if the inner lining of your uterus is still being stimulated by estrogen. If you bleed when you stop taking the progestogen, it indicates estrogen is still being produced by your body and must be "challenged" by progestogen. This process causes the lining to be sloughed off like a menstrual period.

If you are still menstruating but having prolonged or heavy menstrual periods and the tests for cancer are all negative, progestogen may be taken each month to "clean out" the lining of your uterus (called a *chemical D&C*). This will prevent endometrial hyperplasia (thickening of the lining of the uterus which is sometimes a precancerous condition).

- *What will progestogen not do?*

Progestogen will not help vaginal dryness or cracking and alone will not help prevent cardiovascular problems. There is some evidence that progestogen may be helpful in preventing osteoporosis (J. C. Morrison and others, 1980).

- *Birth-control pills increase the risk of blood clots because they contain estrogen. Isn't the same risk there with ERT?*

Birth-control pills contain at least 10 times the amount of estrogen you would receive during estrogen-replacement therapy. The estrogen in ERT—either in the pill form or the transdermal patch has not been shown to affect the clotting factors.[9]

- *What are the advantages of the transdermal (skin-patch) method of taking estrogen?*

1. It is convenient, because it is applied to the abdomen and replaced twice a week.

2. Women are less likely to forget to take it.

3. It has a more constant level of absorption, hence a more constant blood level. Oral estrogen is more likely to give an

9 Lobo, R.A. "Cardiovascular Implications of Estrogen Replacement Therapy." *Obstetrics and Gynecology*. 1990. 75:18S-25S.

"up-and-down" effect.

4. Estrogen delivered in this way does not go directly to the liver (called *first pass*) like oral tablets. This makes it less likely to cause clots, gallstones or elevated blood pressure. It also does not place as much burden upon a damaged liver.

5. Many women who cannot easily tolerate estrogen by mouth can take it as a skin patch. There tends to be less nausea and digestive upset with the skin patch.

6. Because the estrogen in a skin patch avoids the digestive tract, a smaller dose can be given to accomplish the same effect.

- *Several years ago my doctor told me not to take birth-control pills because I was a smoker. He said it would increase the risk of heart attacks and blood clots. Does this same risk exist if I now take estrogen for my hot flashes?*

Birth-control pills contain synthetic estrogens that are 10 to 100 times more potent than the natural estrogens used in ERT. Therefore, they have a much greater impact on clotting factors produced by the liver.

Smoking accelerates coronary atherosclerosis (hardening of the arteries), damages the lining of the blood vessels, activates platelets (helps set clotting process in action), increases the breakdown of estrogen and promotes upper-body fat.[10]

Dr. Claus Christiansen (1985) in Denmark showed smokers had half as much estrogen in their blood as non-smokers taking the same dose of estrogen. We strongly advise you to quit smoking.

- *I am 53 and had thrombophlebitis 10 years ago. When I asked my doctor about taking estrogen to relieve severe menopausal symptoms, she said I should not take it because it would increase the risk of phlebitis again. What am I to do?*

Estrogen is likely to increase the risk of clotting if taken orally. However, if you take your estrogen as a skin patch, the danger is considerably less. You might discuss this possibility with your doctor, but follow her advice because she knows you best.

- *Is it true estrogen increases the chance of high blood pressure and gallstones?*

There is about 1 chance in 20 estrogen could cause release of two

10 Eichner, E.R. "Heart Disease Strikes Women Too." *Your Patient and Fitness.* Oct. 1990. 4:5; 5-11.

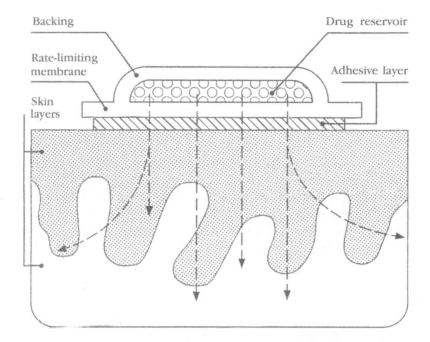

Backing

Drug reservoir

Rate-limiting membrane

Adhesive layer

Skin layers

Cross-section through the Estraderm® skin patch shows construction which allows it to supply estrogen effectively over a several-day period. Arrows indicate path of estrogen being absorbed through the skin and into the bloodstream.

enzymes that cause elevation of blood pressure. But that is true only when the estrogen goes directly to the liver. The skin patch should not do this because the estrogen is absorbed through the skin and does not make a first pass through the liver.

The same applies to gallstones. The skin patch should have practically no effect upon them.

- *Isn't estrogen likely to worsen diabetes?*

You are thinking of birth-control pills. The dose of estrogen is much smaller in ERT. The lower dose used in ERT does not worsen diabetes. Some studies even show an improvement in the diabetes with estrogen use.[11]

- *I have fibroid tumors. Does that mean I can't take estrogen or ERT?*

Fibroids are under the control of estrogen. That's why they

11 Spellacy, W.N. "Menopause, Estrogen Treatment and Carbohydrate Metabolism." *Menopause.* Yearbook Medical Publishers. 1987. 256-258.

decrease in size after menopause when estrogen is no longer produced. However, the low dose of estrogen in ERT is unlikely to stimulate their growth. ETR's advantages outweigh the slight risk of stimulated growth of benign fibroid tumors. If ERT causes your fibroid tumors to increase in size, you can discontinue the therapy.

- *I have a lot of cracking of the skin around my vulva. At times it is so tender I cannot make love. Is this just part of menopause?*

It is normal for the mucous membranes and the skin around the vulva to become thinner and dryer as you become older. This occurs because faltering estrogen levels have lead to a lack of normal lubricating oils in the skin. Consequently, the tissues crack and even bleed. The pain with intercourse is called *dyspareunia*. Contact your doctor to be sure there is no infection and to prescribe estrogen if indicated.[12]

- *How long should I take estrogen if I am taking it to prevent osteoporosis? How much calcium do I need to take with it?*

In general, estrogen seems to have an anti-osteoporotic effect throughout life. Once you have gone through menopause, your ability to absorb calcium may be decreased. You will also require up to 1,000 to 1,600 milligrams of calcium daily to meet your needs—even though you are taking estrogen.

There is a great difference in the various types of calcium and their absorbability. We recommend calcium carbonate which gives you more absorbable calcium in smaller, easier-to-take tablets.

- *Can I take my estrogen as a shot once a month, rather than trying to remember all those pills?*

The biggest problem with a shot is your estrogen level will peak to more than you need, then drop to less than you need. This leaves you over-estrogenated part of the time and underestrogenated the rest of the month. You will have a see-saw, peak-and-valley type blood level of estrogen that may only aggravate your symptoms.

- *Which is better, oral estrogen or patch estrogen?*

The dosage seems to be approximately the same using either

12 Stevenson, J.C. "Pathogenesis, Prevention and Treatment of Osteoporosis." *Obstetrics and Gynecology.* 1990. 75:36S.

method. With patch estrogen your hormone level is more steady and less likely to fluctuate during the day. A patch is only applied twice a week, so you don't have to remember to swallow a pill each day.

Patch estrogen does not make a first pass through the liver and thus avoids some disadvantages of oral estrogen. This is especially favorable if your liver is diseased or if you have had blood clots.

Sensitivity to estrogen can occur with either pill or patch. About 10 percent of women have skin which will not tolerate the patch.

Some women develop nausea, headaches or even rash with the pill form of estrogen.

Cost is slightly greater for patch than for oral estrogen.

- *Do women who have their ovaries removed earlier in life, perhaps in their 30s, require more estrogen to control their menopausal symptoms?*

It appears the earlier in life you have your ovaries removed, the more shocking it is to your body. It may be difficult to regulate the amount of estrogen required to handle the menopausal symptoms. This does not mean menopausal symptoms cannot be controlled if you have your ovaries removed in your 30s. But it does mean your doctor may have a little more difficulty fine-tuning your hormone balance using replacement estrogen and progestogen.

- *If I still have my uterus but have to take estrogen and progestogen, will I begin menstrual periods all over again?*

You might have periods, but they will be light. They should come predictably when you discontinue the progestogen each month. Any bleeding other than this must be reported to your doctor.

It is impossible to discuss the many variations in dosage requirements and the difference in menopausal symptoms. But because there are many estrogen methods and dosages, a program can be devised that is specifically suited to you and your needs. Be patient and give your doctor a chance (months, if necessary) to work out such a program for you.

It may be necessary for you to make several visits to your doctor to have him adjust the dosage or change the medicine. He will need your own input as to how you feel, how you tolerate the estrogen-progestogen program and whether you obtain sufficient relief from troublesome symptoms. He will also need to know if there are any signs of allergy (rashes, etc.) and whether or not you have vaginal bleeding. Together you and your doctor can pilot you through a well-controlled menopause.

- *I heard estrogen will actually make me live longer. Is this true?*

An article in the Journal of the American Medical Association in 1985 stated women on estrogen-replacement therapy tend to live longer, suffer fewer heart attacks and have only one-third the risk of dying from coronary heart disease. Your longevity is lengthened by taking estrogen.

- *My arthritis is definitely worse since going through menopause. A neighbor claims estrogen has helped her arthritis. Is it only psychological?*

As reported in the Journal of the American Medical Association in March 1986, a study in the Netherlands showed the incidence of rheumatoid arthritis is lower in women who are on estrogen-replacement therapy. There is some evidence that pain in this type of arthritis is relieved to some extent when women are on ERT.

Because there are several different types of arthritis, it might depend upon which type you have. Certainly ERT should not make any arthritis worse than it is.

- *I am 47 and just had a D&C which showed I had something called* hyperplasia. *My doctor tells me this is pre-malignant. He wants me to take cyclic progestogen for 3 months. I am frightened to death of cancer. Shouldn't I just have my uterus removed?*

Your doctor is giving you good advice. At the present time you do not have cancer, although endometrial hyperplasia can precede cancer. But your doctor is correct in giving you cyclic progestogen (12 to 13 days each month for 3 months). Your chances of converting the hyperplasia to normal lining are excellent, and this would avoid the need for a hysterectomy.

Your doctor will follow you very closely. He may even take biopsies of the lining of your uterus every few months to make certain it returned to normal. If the endometrial hyperplasia fails to convert to normal, you may have to have a hysterectomy.

- *My doctor insists upon a* baseline mammogram, *as he calls it, before he will start me on estrogen-replacement therapy. Does this mean he suspects cancer of my breast, or is there concern about the relationship of ERT to cancer of the breast?*

ERT does not cause cancer of the breast. However, if you already have cancer of the breast, estrogen may speed up the spread of the cancer. Taking a mammogram lets your doctor rule out the possibility of detectable cancer in your breast.

- *We have a history of heart disease in our family, so I am concerned about cholesterol. I have heard estrogen lowers cholesterol in the blood. Is this so?*

There is desirable cholesterol in the form of HDL (high-density lipoprotein) and undesirable cholesterol in the form of LDL (low-density cholesterol). Estrogen has been shown to raise the level of HDL in the blood. This cholesterol helps prevent plaque formation on the walls of your blood vessels. Also, estrogen appears to have a direct beneficial effect on blood-vessel walls. It appears to keep the smooth muscle in the vessel walls relaxed, which in turn keeps blood pressure down.

This is one possible explanation for the greater protection women have from heart disease before menopause (while their ovaries are still producing estrogen). Within 10 to 15 years after menopause, and without ERT, women have just as many heart attacks as men.

In women under 45 the risk of a heart attack is low. A man has a 40-fold greater risk of having a heart attack. One in 9 women develops cardiovascular disease between 45 and 64. After 65 the risk is 1 in 3.[13]

- *My sister had a hysterectomy along with removal of her ovaries at age 32 because of endometriosis. Does this mean she has a greater risk of heart attack?*

It does unless she is given estrogen-replacement therapy. Within 5 years she will be just as much at risk as men unless she takes estrogen. She should also have ERT combined with calcium to protect her against osteoporosis.

- *My doctor just told me the cause of my bleeding is endometriosis, which he discovered with laparoscopy. What is endometriosis? Is it cancerous?*

The lining of your uterine cavity is called *endometrium.* This is the

13 Eichner, E.R. "Heart Disease Strikes Women Too." *Your Patient and Fitness.* Oct. 1990. 4:5: 5-11.

same lining that is sloughed off and along with some blood makes up your menstrual flow.

When this uterine lining is located somewhere other than where it should be (ovaries, peritoneum, bowel, bladder), the condition is called *endometriosis*. The misplaced tissue may respond to the ovarian hormones each month, continuing to slough off and bleed within the tissues where it is located. Because it bleeds internally, it may cause pain and irritation. These are the characteristic symptoms of endometriosis.

Endometriosis is not cancerous. It only rarely is involved in cancer of the endometrium. Endometriosis is common and may be found in as many as 30 percent of women who have abdominal surgery.

Endometriosis may be relieved by birth-control pills and pregnancy and may be removed by surgery or laser beam. In general, endometriosis is dependent upon your ovaries. When they are removed or cease to function during your menopause, you may expect the symptoms caused by endometriosis to subside.

If you are having symptoms of endometriosis (pain, bleeding) and are near menopause, you can look forward to relief of these symptoms soon. Such a prospect may influence you to defer surgery until you see how much relief you obtain by menopause.

- *I am just starting with menopausal symptoms. I wonder if I should take estrogen because I have varicose veins. Will estrogen increase the risk of blood clots?*

It's OK to take estrogen even though you have varicose veins. The amount of estrogen used to control your menopausal symptoms will not affect your blood-clotting mechanism. This is even more true with the estrogen patch.

If you have a past history of blood clots, we would prescribe estrogen by patch, because the estrogen does not make a first pass through the liver where it might exert some influence on your clotting mechanisms.

- *My hot flashes are unbearable, so I have been taking estrogen along with progestogen. My problem is I also have high blood pressure. I worry about whether the estrogen might make my blood pressure even higher.*

Oral estrogen may cause a release of a substance in the body called *renin*, which can produce a rise in the blood pressure. Estrogen used in ERT generally is tolerated well with little effect

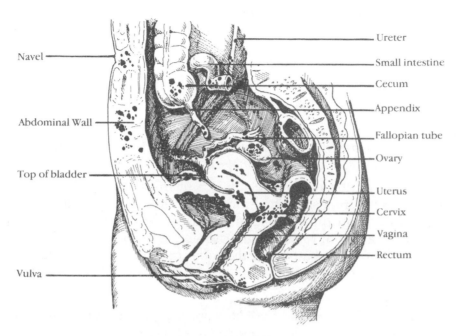

Navel

Abdominal Wall

Top of bladder

Vulva

Ureter

Small intestine

Cecum

Appendix

Fallopian tube

Ovary

Uterus

Cervix

Vagina

Rectum

Sites of endometrial implants.

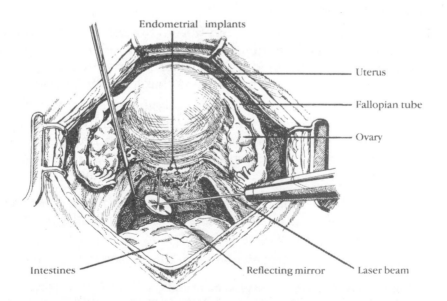

Endometrial implants

Uterus

Fallopian tube

Ovary

Intestines

Reflecting mirror

Laser beam

Vaporization of endometrial implants with a laser beam which can be focused accurately to destroy endometriosis.

on the blood pressure. For those who do get an aggravation of their blood pressure on oral estrogen, we usually prescribe patch estrogen. It does not make a first pass through your liver and is less likely to produce renin and raise your blood pressure.

Recent studies suggest that blood pressure is consistently, although minimally, lowered by estrogen.[14]

- *Recent X-rays showed I have gallstones. A magazine article said estrogen increases the risk of gallstones or at least the pain of a gallstone attack. I also have hot flashes. What can I do for relief?*

Estrogen influences the metabolism of lipids by the liver and increases the cholesterol fraction of bile. This increases the risk of stone formation and gallbladder disease.[15] To avoid this possibility, you may want to take your estrogen as a skin patch. Use the patch if you have had hepatitis (inflammation of your liver) or cirrhosis (when your liver becomes scarred with fibrous tissue).

- *For many years I have had fibroid tumors in my uterus. My doctor has watched them very carefully. Thus far these tumors have not caused any symptoms nor have they increased appreciably in size. Now I am beginning to have severe hot flashes and need some relief. Will estrogen cause these tumors to grow?*

It is true estrogen may cause your fibroid tumors to grow. When fibroid tumors increase in size, they may cause bleeding, pain and pressure on your bladder and other organs. Such a change in size could also indicate a cancerous change in the tumors.

Your doctor can monitor all of these possible effects (there may be none) of estrogen and, if necessary, perform a hysterectomy. Much will depend upon how severe your menopausal symptoms are and how much protection from cardiovascular disease and osteoporosis you want by taking estrogen replacement.

- *I have a friend who drinks a lot of ginseng tea and claims it makes her feel just great. She says it relieves many of her menopausal symptoms. She is encouraging me to try it, but is it safe.?*

Ginseng is a potent estrogen plant. For this reason it helps relieve

14 Hazzard, W.R. "Estrogen Replacement and Cardiovascular Disease, Serum Lipids and Blood Pressure Effects." *American Journal of Obstetrics and Gynecology.* 1989. 161:1847-53.

15 Judd, H.L. "Effects of Estrogen Replacement on Hepatic Function." *Menopause.* Yearbook Medical Publishers. 1987. 237-251.

menopausal symptoms. There are two problems with ginseng:

1. You have no idea how much estrogen you are taking.

2. You are not taking progestogen along with it in cyclic form to protect you against the development of endometrial cancer.

If you are going to take ERT, take it as prescribed and monitored by your doctor *without* ginseng. Leave ginseng to the food faddists. Your friend should do likewise.

- *I am taking estrogen plus progestogen in the form of Provera®. I feel just great while I am taking the estrogen. But when I start the progestogen (last 13 days of the cycle), I feel moody and irritable. My husband suffers as much from my symptoms as I do.*

Not all women tolerate progestogen in the form of Provera®. Sometimes decreasing the dose will help. If this fails to relieve your symptoms, you might try Norlutate® or Micronor®.

We usually start patients on Provera® first, because this drug is less likely to lower the HDL (desirable cholesterol) in your blood.

- *An article I read in the beauty shop said teenagers who have anorexia (loss of appetite) are more likely to develop osteoporosis later in life. I had severe anorexia nervosa as a teenager and now wonder if this will affect me during menopause. I am 47.*

Any woman who experiences significant weight loss during any period in her life and stopped menstruating for 3 months or longer is at great risk of developing osteoporosis. Much depends upon your present status, meaning how much bone mass you have now and whether fractures of your vertebrae (humping of your back, loss of height, etc.) have started.

What you may need at the present time is aggressive treatment with estrogen, calcium and an exercise program to prevent further progression of any osteoporosis. Your doctor may want to get a bone-mineral-density exam to evaluate your current bone mass.

- *I am 46 and still having normal, regular menstrual periods. For the last 4 months I've been experiencing hot flashes. Is this an early menopause? Should I take ERT (estrogen-replacement therapy) to relieve these flashes?*

Menopause often comes on gradually with a decline in estrogen production by your ovaries. Hot flashes can occur off and on during this decline. An FSH (follicle-stimulating hormone) blood test would help us know if ERT would be useful for you.

Often a small dose of estrogen can relieve this discomfort without upsetting your menstrual periods.

- *I'm 51 and have not had a menstrual period for 1-1/2 years. I have no menopause symptoms. Any reason I should take ERT?*

Because you have no symptoms of menopause, there is no reason to prescribe estrogen to relieve symptoms that are not present. But there is another function of estrogen, and that is to prevent osteoporosis and cardiovascular disease. Approximately 1,300,000 to 1,700,000 osteoporosis-related fractures and 650,000 deaths from cardiovascular disease occur each year in post-menopausal women in the United States.

Check with your doctor to see if you have any signs of osteoporosis, including loss of height, curving of your spine, etc. Osteoporosis is a preventable disease and cardiovascular disease can be reduced more than 50%, so talk with your doctor about ERT.

- *I am 53 and have been having increasing anxiety, tension, depression and irritability as well as heart palpitation. I have no hot flashes and do not feel stressed. Are these symptoms related to menopause, even though I don't have hot flashes?*

Even though you do not have hot flashes, your symptoms are very suggestive of estrogen deficiency. See your doctor for ERT and to be sure there are not other underlying medical problems.

- *I am 50 and have some menopausal symptoms. However, I have a strong family history of strokes and heart attacks and worry whether ERT might increase my risk.*

After studying 309 women who had *not* taken estrogen for 5 years in comparison to 301 women who *had* taken estrogen for 5 to 25 years, Dr. Hammond (1984) of Duke University found 28.5 percent new cases of cardiovascular disease in the women who had not taken ERT and only 3.9 percent in those who had.

It appears ERT may offer some protection against hardening of the arteries. Estrogen-replacement therapy is protective and will actually decrease your risk of strokes and heart attacks.

- *Both my parents are being treated for high blood pressure. So far my blood pressure is normal. Will ERT increase my risk of high blood pressure?*

Recent studies showed only 16.3 percent of women on ERT developed high blood pressure as opposed to 31.7 percent of the women who were not taking ERT. The rare occurrence of estrogen-induced hypertension cannot be disputed, but carefully done studies suggest that blood pressure is consistently, although minimally, lowered by ERT.[16] In any event you should be closely followed because of your family history of high blood pressure.

- *At 33 my uterus and ovaries were removed surgically. I have taken ERT ever since. Now I am 55 and my doctor has advised me to discontinue estrogen. I am concerned because I hear women taking ERT live longer than those who don't. Is this true?*

A study reported the overall death rate of women not on ERT for 15 years after surgical menopause was 11.8 percent, whereas the death rate of those on ERT was only 1.4 percent. It appears longevity may be increased in those women who take estrogen after having had their ovaries removed.

There is also the threat of osteoporosis if you discontinue estrogen. Check with your doctor to see if he has other reasons for wanting you to stop taking estrogen.

- *I have been taking estrogen off and on as I felt I needed it. Is there any reason I should not take estrogen this way to relieve my hot flashes, nervousness and insomnia?*

On your "now-and-again" program of estrogen you may develop irregular uterine bleeding and you may cause a build-up of the lining of the uterus (endometrial hyperplasia), which is precancerous. You should be taking a progestogen for 12 days each month with your estrogen. You are also not deriving the full protective effect that continuous, regulated ERT can offer.

Evidence points to consistent use of estrogen as the safest and most effective way to take ERT.

- *Should every woman take estrogen after menopause?*

No! If you are allergic to estrogen, you should not take it.

If you have had an estrogen-related cancer, either breast or uterine, active liver disease or recent deep-vein clots, you should

16 Hazzard, W.R. "Estrogen Replacement and Cardiovascular Disease, Serum Lipids and Blood Pressure Effects." *American Journal of Obstetrics and Gynecology.* 1989. 161:1847-53.

not take it.

With these and perhaps a few other rare exceptions, every woman should take estrogen after menopause to protect against osteoporosis and cardiovascular disease.

- *I've been using the patch for two weeks and I'm having red rings, itchy spots and sometimes red raised areas every place I put the patch. Am I allergic to it?*

Not necessarily. Some women experience this initial irritation the first few weeks, but it usually subsides in a couple of months if they are patient and work with it.

Here are some suggestions on how to manage the skin irritation:

1. Be sure your skin is dry before applying the patch. A hair dryer can be very useful in drying the area where you want to apply the patch.

2. Change the patch location every 12 to 24 hours if you find yourself scratching over the patch or if skin under the patch feels irritated.

3. It is best not to swim, soak in your bath or hot tub with the patch on. Water may seep under the edge and cause further skin irritation. Leave the patch on your vanity and reapply it when your skin is dry.

4. If your patch does not stick (usually after several moves), direct your blow dryer (on HOT) over the patch a few times to warm-up the glue along the edges. It should last the 3-1/2 days.

5. A Benadryl® capsule (25-50mg) or any antihistamine at bedtime can be very helpful in reducing the itching.

6. You may find certain areas of your body tolerate the patch better than others. If so, just rotate the patch site in that area

- *Can I take generic estrogens?*

No! Don't accept substitute generic estrogen because its dosage can vary as much as 25 to 40% compared to brand-name estrogens. You could get a return of symptoms which were well controlled with the brand-name estrogen.

13

Surgery & Menopause

It is never wise to have unnecessary surgery. Risk varies according to the type of surgery, but there is always some risk whenever surgery is performed. For instance, a hysterectomy just to get you through menopause is definitely unwise. The same answer applies when we speak of sterilization. There are simpler and safer methods of sterilization than a hysterectomy. A hysterectomy performed for valid reasons also accomplishes sterilization at the same time.

Surgery is so safe now that it should never be refused when it is necessary.

- *Is any type of surgery more difficult for me to tolerate at the time of menopause? I am thinking of my age, the increased stress at this time and the question of complications.*

We have performed countless female operations and have observed the effects of these and other surgery on our menopausal patients. We have never noticed any delayed healing or any increase in complications in patients just because they were menopausal. Because irregular menstrual flow and often troublesome or uncontrollable uterine bleeding frequently occur as you approach menopause, you may be more likely to require a hysterectomy around 50.

If you require other surgery such as for gallbladder problems, there is no reason you shouldn't have it done just because you are menopausal. We do recommend you understand thoroughly what you are to have done and why. Most doctors have videos or booklets that will explain more about your surgery and answer your questions.

If you understand what is to be done and why, along with any possible complications, you will be better able to cope with surgery. We have also found menopausal women heal just as well as younger women.

- *My nerves seem more fragile since I stopped menstruating a year ago. Any stress upsets me and keeps me from sleeping. Now my doctor wants to remove some intestinal polyps he fears could be malignant. What if the stress throws me into a nervous breakdown?*

If it were elective surgery, you might wait to see if rest and/or some estrogen would help you regain control of your nerves. However, intestinal polyps have a high incidence of malignancy and a high rate of cure if removed early.

Discuss your uneasiness with your doctor. But proceed with biopsy and probable removal of your polyps, even if you are upset emotionally. Your doctor can prescribe mild tranquilizers to relieve your tension if he feels they are necessary.

- *I am scheduled to have an abdominal hysterectomy. My doctor has not suggested my appendix be removed at the same time. Would it increase the risk to any degree to perform an appendectomy at the time as my hysterectomy?*

Although it is true appendicitis is uncommon at your age, it is an easy procedure to remove your appendix while your abdomen is open. It will not increase the risk appreciably, and it will remove the appendix as a threat for future problems.

Adhesions occasionally occur following any abdominal surgery, and they can produce symptoms similar to appendicitis. It is reassuring to know your appendix has been removed and need not be considered when and if you have future abdominal pain.

Are women more likely to have gallstones during menopause?

No. Women are more prone to have gallstones during pregnancy. This is thought to be due to the increased circulating estrogen at that time. There is also a modest relationship between obesity and gallstones. If you gain weight, whether at menopause or otherwise, you may have a greater chance of developing gallstones.

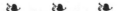

*Many women in midlife experience stress incontinence
(loss of urine when they strain, cough or even laugh).
This can be corrected at the time of hysterectomy.*

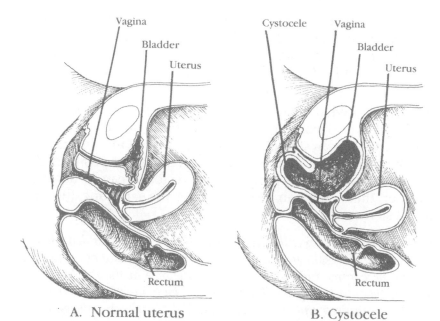

A. Normal uterus

B. Cystocele

A. *Normal uterus, bladder and rectum with good support.*
B. *Cystocele is a hernia of the bladder into the vagina.*

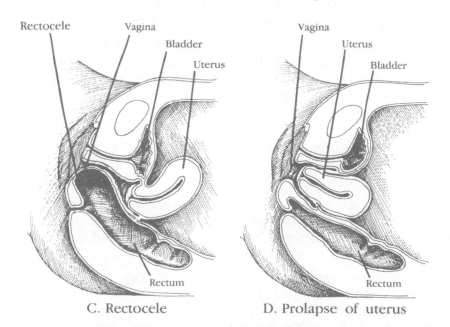

C. Rectocele

D. Prolapse of uterus

C. *Rectocele is a hernia of the rectum into the vagina.*
D. *Beginning prolapse of uterus. Uterus begins to descend into the vagina. You may feel as though "things are falling out."*

- *My problem is rather embarrassing to discuss. When I attempt to have a bowel movement, the stool seems to drop into a pocket in my rectum. This pocket bulges into my vagina. Frequently I must use my thumb to compress this pocket to pass the stool. Can this condition be corrected at the same time I have a hysterectomy?*

Yes. You have what is called a *rectocele,* or a hernia of the rectum into the vagina. This hernia can easily be repaired at the same time as a vaginal hysterectomy. If you have an abdominal hysterectomy, you must then be placed in a different position after (or before) your hysterectomy so your rectocele can be repaired. However, this repair can be done under the same anesthesia as your hysterectomy.

- *I am 47 and have had 5 children. My doctor has recommended I have a hysterectomy. He said my uterus could be removed abdominally or through the vagina and has given me my choice in the matter. I was surprised he didn't simply tell me it should be removed one way or the other. I am confused and do not feel qualified to make that decision.*

There are certain reasons for performing a hysterectomy one way or the other. If your doctor has no preference, then other factors should influence the decision. Usually a surgeon prefers and has been trained more in one method than the other.

The fact you have had 5 children means your vagina probably has been stretched by the births. This makes the vaginal method easier. Because the vagina has been stretched may also mean your vaginal muscles may require tightening—another reason for using the vaginal approach. If the muscles of your vagina (pelvic floor) are tightened, intercourse will be more pleasant for you and your partner. Tightening of the muscles at the time of surgery is accomplished by an incision through the interior posterior vaginal lining. The stretched muscles are then sutured back together.

Do you lose your urine when you cough, sneeze, strain or even laugh? If so, repair of your urethra should be done at the same time as your hysterectomy, whether it is by the abdominal or vaginal route.

If you feel your vagina is too loose for satisfactory intercourse or if you feel as though "things are falling out," your doctor will likely choose the vaginal approach to tighten support of the uterine ligaments and the muscle of your pelvic floor.

Too many women suffer from urinary stress incontinence (involuntary loss of urine due to straining) for years, not realizing this problem can be treated successfully by surgery. Every woman who is going to have a hysterectomy should be asked about this symptom so it can be corrected along with the hysterectomy.

- *I don't see how a doctor can work through such a small opening to remove my uterus through the vagina.*

We mentioned the operation is easier if you have had several children, but it can be done in any case with special instruments and good lighting. In general, we avoid a vaginal approach to a hysterectomy if you have had previous abdominal surgery or if there is a possibility of abdominal adhesions that might prevent your pelvic organs from descending through the vagina.

- *Can my ovaries also be removed through the vagina? I am 48 and do not want to worry about cancer in my ovaries.*

If there are no adhesions, there should be no problem removing your ovaries at the time of vaginal hysterectomy. We agree with you it is better to remove your ovaries along with your uterus at age 48. In fact, serious consideration should be given to removing ovaries, even though they are normal, after age 45.

It is more difficult to remove your ovaries through the vagina, depending on the skill and experience of your surgeon.

- *I have heard recovery time is shorter after a vaginal hysterectomy. Is this true?*

Recovery time may be shorter after a vaginal hysterectomy. If your doctor suggests one particular method over the other, you should go along with his recommendation. He may be more skilled and feel more comfortable performing one type of hysterectomy.

You should, however, talk to him about your bladder, rectum and uterine support and whether or not you require that type of corrective surgery at the same time as your hysterectomy. Risk and post-operative complications are about the same for each method, whether abdominal or vaginal.

- *If I decide to have a vaginal hysterectomy or if my doctor makes this decision, is it likely to be more painful to have intercourse than after an abdominal incision?*

It may take a little longer for your vagina to heal after a vaginal hysterectomy, but healing will occur within 4-6 weeks in either case. If a repair to tighten the vagina was done, your vagina may be more snug and more satisfactory for making love.

- *Are there any advantages to having an abdominal hysterectomy rather than a vaginal hysterectomy?*

  If you have a large uterus, it can be removed more easily through an abdominal incision. If you have had previous abdominal operations or infection involving your pelvic organs, there may be adhesions that would make it difficult to remove your uterus through the vagina.

  An abdominal incision makes it easier to explore your abdominal cavity and inspect all of your other pelvic and abdominal organs, including your appendix and gallbladder. It is worthwhile to know if you have gallstones or whether there are adhesions of the bowel or around your ovaries and tubes (assuming you are not having them removed).

  We have already mentioned we may remove your appendix, even though it is normal. If you ever have abdominal pain in the future, we'll know it is not your appendix. This may save having another operation in the future.

- *Can you summarize the advantages and disadvantages of abdominal versus vaginal hysterectomy?*

  Advantages of Abdominal Hysterectomy:

  - Permits complete exploration of abdominal organs and removal of appendix.
  - Permits easier, less time-consuming surgery in difficult cases in which there are adhesions, large tumors or other problems.
  - Less risk of infection in post-operative period.

  Disadvantages of Abdominal Hysterectomy:

  - Abdominal scar is visible and may be unsightly or painful.
  - Longer recovery time.
  - Occasional hernia through incision.
  - Increased risk of adhesions (bowel sticking to bladder or incision).

  Advantages of Vaginal Hysterectomy:

  - No visible scar and no hernia of incision.
  - Shorter hospital stay and recovery time.

ஃ Less operation time and shorter anesthesia time.

ஃ Less chance of gas pains and bowel adhesions.

ஃ Less post-operative pain and fewer analgesics needed.

ஃ Better for high-risk patients.

ஃ Enables surgeon to repair bladder (cystocele), bowel (rectocele) and uterine prolapse.

Disadvantages of Vaginal Hysterectomy:

ஃ Cannot explore abdominal organs.

ஃ Difficult to remove large tumors.

ஃ Cannot remove ovaries and tubes when bound by adhesions.

ஃ May shorten vagina for intercourse.

ஃ More post-operative infections.

- *A friend of mine was given some exercises to tighten her vagina and they seem to be working. What kind of exercises would these be? Would they avoid the necessity of surgery to correct loss of vaginal support?*

Several decades ago Dr. Arnold H. Kegel developed what have come to be known as *Kegel Exercises* to strengthen muscles in the pelvic floor and improve control during intercourse. There are two exercises.

1. Tighten or squeeze your vagina and your rectum by drawing these muscles up into the vagina. Squeeze your buttocks together and hold in this position for 5 to 10 seconds. Then relax and repeat the exercise as many times as you can, gradually working up to 100 or more times each day.

This exercise can be performed at any time and in any position, because no one will be aware you are exercising. You can do it while sitting at a desk, standing at your sink or whatever.

2. As you pass your urine, practice starting and stopping the stream as many times as you can. This exercise will strengthen the muscles around your urethra and give you better control over your bladder. If your stress incontinence is not too severe and if you persist in this exercise, you may find your control will improve so surgical repair is no longer necessary.

- *What is the risk in hysterectomy?*

The mortality rate in hysterectomy is about 2 per 1,000

operations. The risk varies, of course, with your age, your general health and the skill of your physician, among other things.

- *My sister just had a hysterectomy. Her incision was almost completely concealed in her pubic hair. Why is the incision made there?*

Although some women prefer to have a Pfannenstiel (also called the *bikini incision*) so they can wear a bikini without their scar being obvious, the principal reason for using this type of abdominal incision is to obtain better support post-operatively. Such an incision heals better, faster, with less pain and practically never pulls apart (ruptures).

A Pfannenstiel incision is a semicircular (moon-shaped) incision that is mostly, if not completely, concealed by your pubic hair. It generally heals with a smaller, almost-invisible scar because it follows natural creases. This incision takes somewhat longer to make and to repair, but it looks better cosmetically. As mentioned above, it will provide better support post-operatively.

If you have had a previous vertical incision from your pubic hairline extending upward to your navel, we usually cut out this scar and continue the vertical incision through the skin. Under the skin, the same muscles and fasciae must be separated along anatomical lines in both the vertical and the Pfannenstiel incisions.

- *If I have a problem controlling my urine, can this problem be corrected through an abdominal incision at the same time I have an abdominal hysterectomy?*

Yes. In most cases your urethra (rather than your bladder) can be repaired through an abdominal incision. You may want to discuss this with your doctor and make certain he is aware you have urinary stress incontinence.

- *If my uterus is being removed because of cancer, can my problem of stress incontinence also be treated at the same time?*

Yes. Correction of urinary stress incontinence by *urethropexy,* as it is called, can be carried out without any significant increase in risk. In most instances in which urinary stress incontinence and terminal constipation (due to rectocele) are not corrected during a hysterectomy operation, either your doctor has not inquired about these symptoms or you have not complained about them.

It is important to know these problems can be corrected at the

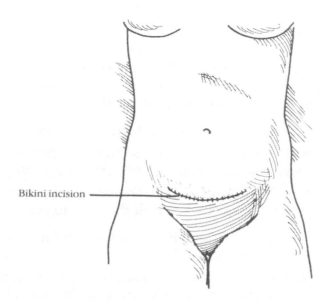

Bikini incision

"Bikini" incision (Pfannensteil) is a transverse eliptically shaped incision made within the hairline where it does not show. Surgically, it gives better post-operative support than a vertical incision.

time you have a hysterectomy. Discuss them with your doctor *before* your surgery.

- *My vagina has seemed loose since I had my four children. My babies were large and I feel I was stretched too much during labor and delivery. It is especially noticeable when we make love. Can anything be done about this problem during my hysterectomy?*

Your vagina can be repaired by tightening the stretched muscles of your vagina and pelvic floor during a vaginal hysterectomy through the same incision.

If you have an abdominal hysterectomy, these same muscles can be repaired, but it requires that you be repositioned on the operating table after your abdominal incision has been repaired. You are re-scrubbed and re-draped to perform the repair. This separate operation will prolong the operating and anesthesia time. But it can be done under the same anesthesia and will save you another trip to the hospital to have this repair done later. There is minimal, if any, increase in risk to include such a repair with your hysterectomy.

- *What if I should decide to have a vaginal hysterectomy and then my doctor finds adhesions or some other problem that makes removal of my uterus through the vagina impossible. What happens then?*

You are simply repositioned on the operating table, re-scrubbed and re-draped for an abdominal incision and the operation is completed as though it had been planned that way.

- *How soon will I be able to resume sex relations after my hysterectomy?*

We recommend you wait 4 to 6 weeks after your hysterectomy whether it is performed abdominally or through your vagina.

Caution is advised, but generally you should have no discomfort while making love if you give yourself this time to heal.

- *Are you sure having my uterus or my ovaries removed will not affect my desire or my ability to have sex?*

From an anatomical or physiological aspect, there is no reason for you to find any difference in libido or orgasm after a hysterectomy or other surgery. If you had a normal sex life before surgery, you should have a normal response after surgery. The same applies to a man who has a vasectomy.

But there are women who feel they have been defeminized somehow. This mistaken idea has a negative psychological effect upon their love making. Discuss your feelings with your doctor before you have surgery. Your attitude will have much to do with the way you respond after your hysterectomy.

- *I was surprised to learn there are different types of hysterectomy. Some hysterectomies put you through the change and others do not. Can you clarify this?*

Surgical menopause is explained on page 17, but let us say once again: *The uterus has nothing to do with menopause.* Menopause has to do with your ovaries and estrogen production.

A simple hysterectomy in which only the uterus is removed will stop your menstrual periods because you have no uterus from which to bleed. It will prevent you from becoming pregnant, because you have no place in which to carry a pregnancy.

But a simple removal of your uterus (hysterectomy) will not cause menopausal symptoms such as hot flashes, nervousness and the many other changes that occur when the ovaries stop functioning and estrogen production ceases. Confusion arises because ovaries are often removed along with the uterus, thus causing surgical menopause.

Surgical removal of the ovaries causes an abrupt end to estrogen production by your ovaries. This causes instant menopause unless you are given replacement hormones (estrogen and progestogen). The symptoms can be shocking and severe. For this reason your doctor will place you immediately after surgery on replacement hormones (estrogen and progestogen). This usually prevents any noticeable change due to loss of your ovaries.

Every woman is different and may require a different amount of hormones to alleviate or prevent menopausal symptoms. A period of "fine tuning" may be necessary to establish the exact dose of estrogen-progestogen that is best suited to your needs. As stated on page 73, it is also possible you might require a small dose of testosterone, the male sex hormone, to help balance your needs. Your doctor can determine what you need, but it may take some time.

Many women do not need a hysterectomy or any surgery at the time of menopause. But those women who do have these operations can do so with confidence that they will feel better afterward. We now have hormones and other medicines to prevent the symptoms that used to plague women who had surgery at this time in life.

಄ ಄ ಄

A hysterectomy is not defeminizing.

14

Cosmetic Surgery & Menopause

Whether or not cosmetic surgery is right for you depends to some extent on the way your perceive yourself. You may prefer to just be yourself and let the chips fall where they may. You may be so busy you are not concerned with how you look. Perhaps you accept the changes that accompany aging as part of life and get on with it.

Sometimes, because of exposure to the public in your profession as an actress, performer, politician, business executive, etc., or just for personal self-esteem, you may feel a need to improve your appearance and reverse some of the changes age imposes upon you. Regardless of the reason, you need to know what can and cannot be accomplished by modern cosmetic surgery.

Be sure to discuss thoroughly with your doctor just what you expect from your cosmetic surgery. If you have unrealistic expectations, you could end up disappointed. It is wrong for your doctor to mislead you by *permitting* you to expect more than the surgery can deliver.

Give yourself plenty of time to consider all aspects of the surgery. Write down all of your questions and insist upon answers to these questions. Keep in mind the aging process continues and surgical cosmetic changes will last for only a few years.

- *At 52 I am finally through menopause. My children are married and now I have time for myself. I've watched the skin on my neck and upper lip become wrinkled and would like to do something about it. How safe is face-lift surgery?*

Gravity may have its many advantages, but one of them is not the effect it has on your facial skin. Just how much sagging and wrinkling there is seems to depend upon the genes you inherit and how much fatty tissue you have lost from beneath your skin. Whether you accept your fate or want to change it depends upon

195

your attitude toward modern cosmetic surgery.

With the many improvements in technique, this type of surgery is safe and successful. Many plastic surgeons perform this type of surgery under local anesthesia in their own offices and surgical suites. Face-lift surgery is rather costly. With few exceptions, your insurance will not underwrite this kind of surgery.

- *If I do not have to be hospitalized for face-lift surgery, how long will I have to miss work?*

Much depends upon whether or not you are exposed to the public. Your surgeon can discuss with you how much surgery you will require and how extended your recovery will be. A classic face lift involves your cheeks, neck, jowls and the skin on the outer part of your eyelids. It may also involve your forehead.

Face-lift surgery involves extensive undermining of tissues which will leave them bruised and discolored. To remove wrinkles from your upper lip may require sanding or a chemical peel of the tissues, which leaves them traumatized.

Face-lift surgery is both common and safe.

- *Is there any way I might know whether a face lift will help me?*

There is a simple test you can perform to give you a general idea whether a lift will help you. Stand in front of your mirror and use your fingers to lift the tissues on the sides of your face just in front of your ears. See illustration. Although not completely accurate, it does give you an idea of what can be accomplished by face-lift surgery.

- *I have heard there are other methods besides a face lift that will remove wrinkles.*

You may be thinking about a *chemical peel.* A chemical is applied that causes the outer layers of skin to peel away. This leaves the underlying tissues to heal by scarring, which removes some of the wrinkles in its wake. *Dermabrasion* is another process in which wrinkles and acne scars are removed by sanding your skin just like sanding the rough spots out of a piece of wood.

One of the newer methods for improving the appearance of your skin involves the injection of collagen under your skin to replace the fatty tissue that has been lost. Although collagen fills out your skin and irons out the wrinkles from the inside, so to speak, it is eventually absorbed in certain women and may disappear after

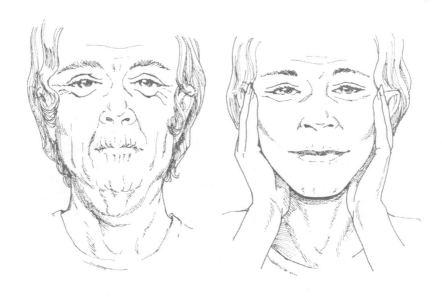

Patient's test for what a face lift might accomplish. This test is partially accurate, but wrinkles around lips and nose will remain to some degree. Jawline and neck will be improved the most.

a few months.

Cosmetic surgery can remove bags from under your eyes and correct sagging eyelids. Whether or not you choose to have any of these procedures done may depend upon their importance to you and the size of your pocketbook.

- *Is it likely my face lift will have to be repeated every few years?*

    Aging will continue until you die. Although a face lift is longer acting in some than in others, you should plan on a gradual return of your wrinkles and sagging over a period of 2 to 5 years. A face lift is not a total problem-solver. You still must accept yourself and your aging.

    A frank discussion with your surgeon may establish that a face lift is definitely for you, or you may find a more suitable alternative.

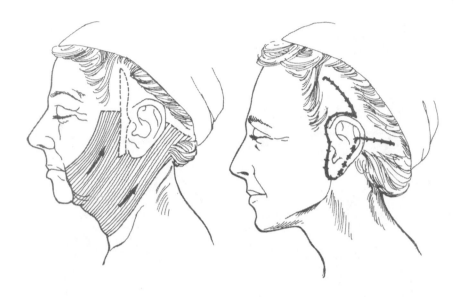

Shaded area shows skin that must be dissected free to pull skin tight to decrease wrinkles. Excess skin is removed in triangles above and on either side of the ear.

- *In spite of rigid dieting and the fact I am not overweight for my height, I still have a bulging, sagging tummy. How safe and effective is a tummy-tuck operation?*

Women have this problem more often than men, because their abdomen is stretched during pregnancy. Sometimes your abdominal muscles regain their tone, but leave sagging, over-stretched skin that protrudes to show bulges under your clothing unless rigidly controlled by a girdle.

If the bulging involves skin only, the excess skin can be easily and safely removed, usually as an outpatient or in your doctor's surgical suite, under local anesthesia. If the underlying muscles and support fascia (thick, gristly-like tissue that extends between muscles to give support) have stretched beyond what exercising can correct, a more extensive operation must be undertaken.

Let's admit it. Our particular culture worships thinness. Women are expected to be thin and to have flat stomachs. In certain other cultures these same women would be judged undesirable and ill-nourished.

Present-day fashions are not designed for women with a protruding tummy! If you have already resorted to a muumuu-type dress, a tummy-tuck operation may be for you. Talk to your doctor about this operation if you have already tried exercise and diet and have failed to get rid of that sagging stomach.

- *How safe is a tummy-tuck operation?*

This operation is much safer than it used to be. It is performed far more often than years ago, simply because it is demanded more by modern society. If your muscles also must be tightened, your surgery is more complex and carries a greater risk. It may demand hospitalization, general anesthesia and more prolonged hospitalization. See illustration, page 200.

A tummy-tuck operation may be done at the same time you have other abdominal surgery, such as a hysterectomy. This is something you may want to discuss with your gynecologist or surgeon before you have your operation. It does require a plastic surgeon.

Sometimes your bulging tummy is due to an actual rupture (hernia) of the supporting tissues of your lower abdomen and would then require more extensive repair of these tissues. Any operation entails some risk. This fact should be considered before you make your decision concerning surgery.

- *From my waist up I look fairly normal and am satisfied with my appearance. But despite my best efforts at dieting, my hips bulge and seem all out of proportion to my upper torso. Can anything be done to correct the dilemma?*

You are not alone. Many women find all attempts at weight loss simply result in smaller breasts and a thin, haggard look in their face, with no apparent loss of weight in their hips. Despite claims to the contrary, exercise will not cause you to lose weight in specific areas of your body. You lose it all over, mostly in the areas where you carry the most weight. To "spot-reduce" you need to exercise a specific area to tighten and tone the muscle underneath.

ès   ès   ès

Discuss thoroughly with your doctor what cosmetic surgery can and cannot do for you. "Before" and "after" pictures of other patients may help. You should also realize a face lift may have to be repeated in a few years because the aging process goes on.

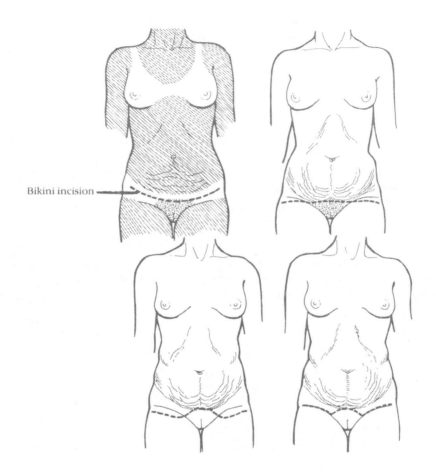

Bikini incision

Incisions used for tummy-tuck surgery. "Bikini" type is indicated. Other incisions are variations used according to the distribution of fat and the preference of the surgeon.

Until recent years, surgery had nothing to offer to correct this situation. Now *subcutaneous suction lipectomy* can help. The excess amount of fat that occurs in wavy ripples under your skin, the excess-fatty-tissue health radicals love to call *cellulite*, can now be removed by a new type of surgery.

Suction lipectomy is called *fat-suctioning, suction-assisted lipectomy, lipo-dissection* and a few other medical terms. In reality this surgery is a type of spot-reduction but this term smacks of quackery, which suction lipectomy is not. "Lipo" means fat and "ectomy" means getting rid of it, whether it is by cutting, suctioning or by some other method.

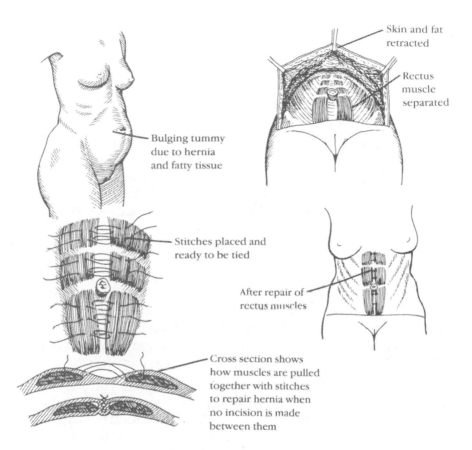

Skin and fat
retracted

Rectus
muscle
separated

Bulging tummy
due to hernia
and fatty tissue

Stitches placed and
ready to be tied

After repair of
rectus muscles

Cross section shows
how muscles are pulled
together with stitches
to repair hernia when
no incision is made
between them

*Repair of an abdominal hernia (diastasis recti) can be carried out at the
same time you have a hysterectomy.*

Suction lipectomy seems to be here to stay. The various methods
are constantly improving both as to technique and safety. It can
be done as an outpatient or in your doctor's operating suite,
usually with local anesthesia, unless the area to be reduced is too
extensive.

- *How is suction lipectomy actually accomplished?*

Through small, 1/4- to 1-inch incisions, your doctor uses a tiny
wand or suction dissector attached by a tubing to a high-powered
suction machine to remove the fat. See page 204. As with any
surgery, rigid sterile technique must be used to avoid infection.

Prior to surgery your plastic surgeon marks on your skin the definite areas from which you wish to have excess fatty tissue removed. He will discuss with you ahead of time how extensive the surgery will be and how much fat you want removed.

Although the incision is tiny, the area covered by the suction wand is rather large. By a series of long parallel strokes, the fat is methodically removed. It is important to leave columns of undisturbed tissue between the strokes to preserve blood supply and to promote healing.

Because of the particular method of fat removal, you must realize the result may reveal some unevenness. Pressure dressings are used to attempt to give a smooth result. In general, your surgeon might err on the side of removing too little fatty tissue rather than too much, realizing he can always remove more tissue at a later time if necessary.

- *What are the risks of suction lipectomy?*

Risks become even more important because suction lipectomy is strictly cosmetic surgery. Cosmetic surgery is performed not out of necessity but to improve appearance. Any surgery involves risks of anesthesia, infection and allergic reactions. You have the additional risk of your own response to surgery. Your age, the texture of your skin and its elasticity must be considered.

Unwanted dimpling of your skin may occur, or you may find some unsightly edges surrounding the areas that have been removed. You may also have to undergo additional surgery to accomplish exactly the result you and your surgeon desire. Techniques are steadily improving as well as the results.

Sensory changes vary from itching, tingling, hypersensitivity and numbness. Most symptoms disappear in 6 to 12 months. Swelling, bruising and occasional prolonged discomfort are possible complications along with a rare hematoma (pocketing of blood).

Uncommon is the risk of a blood clot or a globule of fat that escapes into the blood stream. Unlikely but possible is a slough of some of the skin that has been undermined. This is why parallel-yet-separated strokes as the fat is removed might produce unevenness. A pressure dressing must be tight enough to prevent bleeding without shutting off circulation.

Much of the success of this operation depends on your attitude and self-image. Suction lipectomy may produce a marked difference in your appearance, but it can't change your self-image or your self-esteem. Those you must change by yourself.

Suction lipectomy is not a way to lose weight. It is designed to change the your appearance, but it can't contour of your body and remove undesirable fat that remains although you've lost weight from other areas of your body. If you regain excessive weight in your body after suction lipectomy, expect fat to return to some of these same areas of your body. Removal of the fat cells does help prevent this return of fat.

Suction lipectomy is a very successful and satisfying operation when it is wisely applied. It can "spot-reduce" you as no other procedure or program can. It may be just the operation you need as you change your image during menopause.

- *I have had 5 children. It seems as though each child has taken part of my breasts with it. I literally have no breasts left, and what is left hangs like a loose piece of skin.*

Now you have decided upon a new image, you certainly can order the size and contour you want in your breasts. Surgery in which your breasts are enlarged is called *augmentation mammaplasty*. It is common. More than 100,000 such operations were performed in 1987, most of them right in the doctor's office. Realistically we think far more mammaplasties than this were performed, because it is difficult to keep track of operations done in doctors' suites.

Augmentation mammaplasties involve several procedures, depending upon the size and shape of your breast to begin with. If your breasts are too pendulous, some of the skin tissue must be removed. If your breasts are large enough but have sagged, the nipple can be relocated by any one of several techniques at the same time your breast is reconstructed.

Most cases involve inserting a plastic envelope which contains saline solution into your breast to give the size and contour you desire.

- *Do breast implants really feel like breasts, or are they merely for appearance?*

Years ago a mammaplasty was uncommon and often unsatisfactory. The implant frequently caused a tissue reaction and eventually hardened so it felt more like a cantaloupe than a breast. Modern breast prostheses cause little tissue reaction and really do have the consistency of a breast.

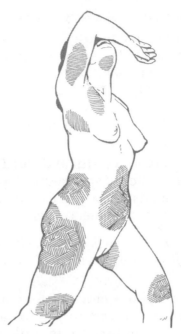

Shaded areas show places where fat will be removed during suction lipectomy. Hips and abdomen are most frequently involved in this surgery.

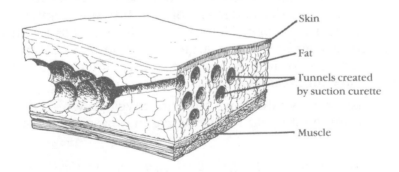

Suction Lipectomy: By tunneling with a suction curette, enough blood supply is left intact to ensure rapid healing. Tunnels are less likely to permit hematomas.

- *Can I really have the size breasts I want? My breasts are small, almost like a man's. I am very sensitive about it.*

It is true, within the limitations of your skin-stretchability. You can have the size breasts you want by implanting that particular size prosthesis. Before you demand extremes, however, you should consider a few factors. You may not want the additional weight of heavier breasts. Heavy breasts sometimes are difficult to support and may cause backache.

The size of your breasts will influence the way you must dress, the styles you must select and the gawks and stares you may provoke. Don't order a size prosthesis that is out of proportion to your body size. Although your doctor can replace your present prosthesis with a smaller one or a larger one in another expensive operation, try to choose the size with which you will be permanently happy.

- *What are the risks and possible complications of augmentation mammaplasty?*

In addition to the risks of any surgery, there's always the possibility of infection, hematoma (accumulation of blood in a pocket) and some loss of sensation in your nipple. Nipple-numbness occurs in about 15 percent of women. It's usually temporary, but it can be permanent. This may be important if you depend upon nipple stimulation as part of sexual arousal when you make love.

Hardening of the implant occurs in 10 to 15 percent of women. It may result in the formation of a fibrous capsule surrounding the implant. This capsule is more common when the implant is placed under the fatty tissue of your breast rather than when it is placed under the muscles that underlie your breast. See pages 207–208. This hardening is troublesome and discouraging, because it takes away much of the normal "feel" of your new breast.

Talk to your surgeon about this possible complication before you have the surgery so you will be informed about the condition. Repeat surgery can often correct and relieve this hardening. But a completely satisfactory soft breast may be difficult to achieve once fibrosis (scarring) has occurred.

The capsule surrounding your artificial breast may rupture or leak, but this is uncommon. Leaking demands repeat surgery with the insertion of another implant. Only rarely does the implant slip or slide into a position in which your breast appears lopsided, but the condition must be corrected surgically.

The scarring following initial surgery may also make re-align-
ment and repositioning of the implant envelopes difficult.

Augmentation mammaplasty has been a godsend to women with
flat chests. It has given them a self-esteem no other procedure or
any amount of counseling could have done. Keep it in mind if you
are not satisfied with your present lack of breast contour.

- *My problem is different. I have always been plagued by heavy,*
  uncomfortable, large breasts that give me backache and defy any
  brassiere to support them. Now I am in menopause they have become
  even larger, despite the fact I have not gained any weight otherwise.

It is true some women notice a tremendous increase in the size of
their breasts during menopause or thereafter. It is too bad breast
size can not be averaged out to make everyone happy.

In your own case, it is unfortunate you were not offered an
operation called *reduction mammaplasty* many years ago. Women
as early as their late teens have been operated upon to correct this
same problem. One 18-year-old patient of ours had large, atten-
tion-provoking breasts that were entirely out of proportion to her
petite figure. It was gratifying to see her delight at being what she
considered "normal" again and not subject to unkind and inap-
propriate remarks wherever she went. The operation relieved her
backache and the pain from bra straps cutting into her shoulders.
It also simplified her shopping for dress styles.

- *How safe is reduction mammaplasty?*

Any surgery involves some risk. But reduction-mammaplasty
techniques are safe and sensible.

The overall complication rate for reduction mammaplasty is
about 25 percent. A few of these complications are serious; most
are not. Only a small number of these complications seriously
affect the desired result, while the others have no effect upon the
final outcome of surgery.

Because of the amount of tissue that must be dissected, the most
common complication is a hematoma, in which blood accumu-
lates in a pocket within the breast. As you might guess, it is
difficult to use a very tight pressure dressing over the breast. Even
meticulous surgery can be complicated by post-operative bleeding.

If the hematoma is small, it will be absorbed and can be left alone.
If it is large, it will have to be drained.

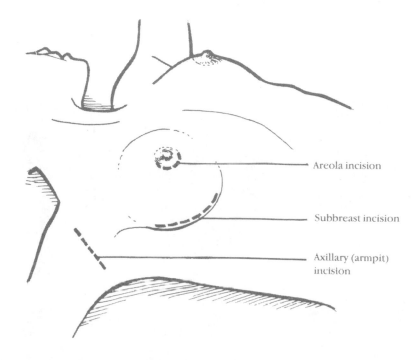

Areola incision

Subbreast incision

Axillary (armpit) incision

Augmentation Mammaplasty: Three potential incision sites through which saline-filled envelopes can be inserted into breast.

If bleeding in the breast persists, the wound has to be re-opened so the bleeding blood vessel can be tied off. If sufficient tissue is undermined by the hematoma, it can cause sloughing of the relocated nipple along with considerably more scarring.

If the relocated nipple sloughs away, the deformity is permanent. Although such a deformity is not visible through your clothing, it may be difficult for you to accept cosmetically, possibly because of sexual implications.

Sometimes the relocated nipple retracts or becomes otherwise deformed. Sometimes it is simply mislocated at the time of surgery. You may notice some loss of sensation in your breast. If you have a tendency to form keloids (unsightly scars), you may be unhappy about the appearance of your scar.

But overall, the most grateful patients we have are those who have had reduction mammaplasties. Their most frequent comment has

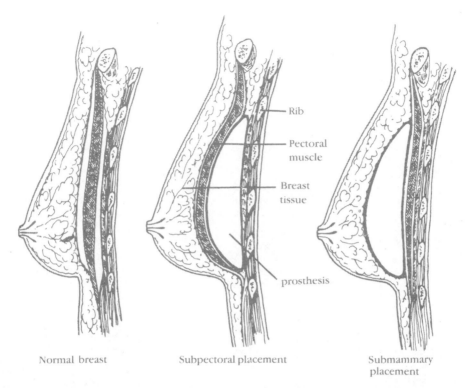

Normal breast   Subpectoral placement   Submammary placement

Rib

Pectoral muscle

Breast tissue

prosthesis

Breast augmentation with a saline-filled envelope placed between the breast and pectoral muscle or under the pectoral muscle.

been, "Why didn't someone tell me about this sooner?" Their relief from backache and from the discomfort of cutting bra straps is immeasurable.

• *How is this remarkable reduction in breast tissue accomplished—especially to obtain an attractive breast contour post-operatively?*

This is best described with an illustration. You can see from the drawing how the excess breast tissue is removed and the nipple is relocated. Your plastic surgeon must determine where and how much to cut and how much tissue to leave. The test for success of the operation is how satisfied you are with the end result.

Isn't it great to know something can be done to help you?

One of the most important things for you to realize is cosmetic surgery cannot perform miracles. It is possible it cannot do all

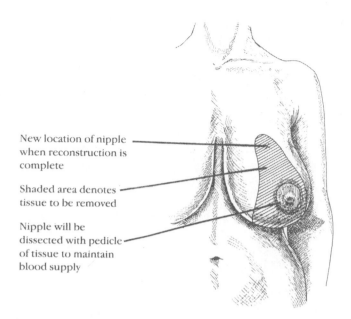

New location of nipple when reconstruction is complete

Shaded area denotes tissue to be removed

Nipple will be dissected with pedicle of tissue to maintain blood supply

Reduction Mammaplasty: The breast is carefully measured by the doctor and the new location for the nipple is determined. Shaded area shows amount of tissue to be removed.

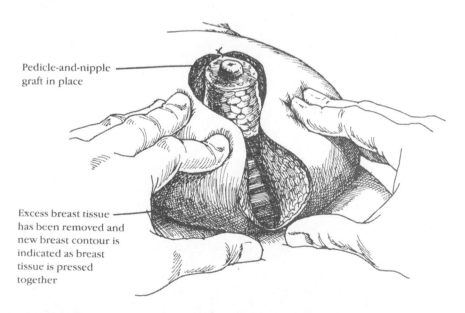

Pedicle-and-nipple graft in place

Excess breast tissue has been removed and new breast contour is indicated as breast tissue is pressed together

A wedge of breast tissue has been removed, cutting around the pedicle graft of the nipple. The nipple has been anchored in place at its new location.

you expect or would like to see happen. Be sure to discuss any cosmetic surgery thoroughly with your plastic surgeon before the operation. Feel free to ask any questions that trouble you.

Your doctor will probably take pictures before and after so you can compare the results. An informed patient is more likely to be a happy one.

15

Aging & Menopause

Fifty is merely a chronological age. Your true age is how you feel about yourself. You have probably already come to the realization that aging has a lot to do with your attitude toward reaching another milestone each year.

It is true some people age faster in their appearance than others, no matter what kind of care they take of themselves. Heredity smiles on some with a smooth, wrinkle-free skin and a pain-free, agile body while bequeathing arthritis, diabetes, high blood pressure and wrinkles on others.

So, you ask, is there anything you can do to slow down whatever Nature has given you as your lot in the last one-third of your life? Yes, at 50 you still have about one-third of your life ahead of you and probably more (perhaps 34 years). Begin by deciding you are going to:

1. Enjoy every day of the life you have ahead of you.

2. Reflect happiness to those around you. One patient just celebrated her 83rd birthday and was so excited about it and so appreciative of the attention that all of us enjoyed it as much as she did. This woman is one of the most pleasant individuals we have ever seen and a pure delight to be around. All of this is despite a severe fall resulting in a fractured hip along with several other disabilities.

Another 80-year-old patient in excellent physical health is so negative that the only way she can brighten a room is to leave it. Despite having nearly everything life can offer in the way of comfort, she takes a dim view of every comment, every kindness and even the love that is offered to her. Because of her negative attitude, she drives well-intentioned friends and relatives away. Then she complains of loneliness.

3. Search for ways to give service to others. If you want to forget your own problems, help others overcome theirs. You soon discover everyone has a satchel-full of problems. Although these problems vary somewhat in weight, each individual must develop her own muscles to carry them. Be one of those who helps carry her neighbor's burdens.

One depressed, menopausal, 49-year-old patient found a new life and quickly forgot her own worries when she became a volunteer in a nearby hospital. Another 56-year-old lost her menopausal symptoms when she volunteered at a children's hospital as a "love mother," an assignment in which she held infants and small children on her lap and loved them.

We have no statistics to prove this, but we think you will actually feel younger when you are giving of yourself to help others.

4. Maintain a lively interest in things that are going on. One reliable sign of aging, even premature aging, is a tendency constantly to reminisce about the past instead of discussing current events. Most young people are "now" oriented. They are concerned with what is going on around them today. And they quickly lose interest when you talk to them about the "good old days."

Read your newspapers and watch the TV news. Know what is going on in the world. Reserve your reminiscing for those instances when you are requested to talk about them.

5. Turn each conversation away from yourself and direct it upon the person with whom you are speaking. If you want to be known as a brilliant and delightful conversationalist, be an attentive listener.

6. Explore new areas of learning. One woman at 65 took a night class in art, something she had never done before. In the same college she progressed to sculpting. When she died at 86 she was known as one of the finest sculptors in the entire area.

7. Growing older gracefully includes growing older gratefully. Be thankful at 50 that you have a lot of time ahead of you to investigate fields of knowledge you have never had an opportunity to enter before. Wouldn't it be exciting to discover you have an undiscovered, entirely new talent?

8. If you still feel you want a "physical" change, re-read Chapter 14 on Cosmetic Surgery & Menopause.

- *I read that a woman who lives to be 50 has another third of her life ahead of her, which would mean 75. Yet in a recent article the expected age was said to be 85. Which is correct?*

Recent statistics show a woman who lives to be 50 and is in good health may live to be 92! This is good news to the more than 35-million women who are over age 50 in the United States.

- *Within 5 years I will have the option of retiring, at which time I will be 55. Right now I have no plans for retirement. Will retirement make me age faster?*

In general, retirement should mean retiring *to* something else you perhaps enjoy more, find less stressful, more challenging and something that will give you more satisfaction than your present job. If you cannot find something more satisfying than your work to occupy your time and your mind when you retire, perhaps you should consider staying where you are. You will definitely age faster if you have nothing to do and may die of boredom at any age, even though you aren't buried until later.

Some studies have shown memory remains sharper if you continue to use it. Your alertness, attention span and ability to solve problems will maintain a higher level if you are required to use these skills. Plan now for new interests for your retirement, or you may find you will quickly age to 75 or 80 in a few short years.

- *At 65 I was forced to retire. But I still feel well, enjoy good physical and mental health and would like to continue to work. I still feel I have much to contribute in the working world. What are your suggestions?*

Interestingly many companies have now begun to rehire some of these retirees. They find older people are more mature, more reliable in most instances, take fewer sick days and have much to contribute because of their experience. Older people are also less demanding. You might want look for such a company.

Many older women are returning to college and consistently find their grades in the upper curves, often at the top. You are less distracted than those students who are 30 or so years younger than yourself. Your maturity more than makes up for their quick-wittedness. You are never too old to learn—quite the contrary. We congratulate you on your desire to continue working.

Remember you are not as young in some ways as you used to be. Every year nearly 20 percent of all people over 65 suffer serious falls. Falls are the leading cause of accidents in this age group.

- *I am 52 and have never been an exerciser. Yet I find myself with a sincere desire to become more physically fit and see if I can't get my body into shape. Is it too late and would it be damaging to my body to undertake an exercise program at this late date?*

You are never too old to start exercising, but you may have to be more cautious. Your body probably will require a longer time to adapt to exercise. First of all, check with your doctor to make certain there is no reason you shouldn't exercise.

Before undertaking a sports program, get yourself in shape by following the instructions in Chapter 9 on Fitness & Menopause. But by all means get started as soon as possible. Exercise *will* help slow down the aging process if it is done sensibly.

- *When I look at my body in profile in the mirror, I look old! Yet I am only 49. My back arches in a hump around my shoulders and my tummy protrudes. What can I do?*

Begin by improving your posture. Try standing at attention as though you were in the Armed Forces. Throw your shoulders back, your head up and your chest out. Immediately you will notice an improvement in your back and bustline. Pulling your chin in and your chest out helps to avoid humping forward, a stance too often characteristic of middle-agers.

Now pull in your stomach and wear a belt tight enough so it reminds you to hold your stomach in.

Try to be aware of good posture all the time. It really is possible to change your posture after all these years of slumping! Even though osteoporosis may have produced some irreversible humping of your back, some of this is due to poor posture. It is this "correctible humping" you want to change. As you progress further into your exercise program, you may find your posture will also improve, simply because your muscles become stronger.

- *Are there any foods that will slow down aging of my body?*

If you are thinking of appearance, there are no foods that will make any difference despite some advertising claims to the contrary. Healthwise you should follow a well-balanced diet.

- *I am 54 and have smoked 2 packs of cigarettes a day for at least 35 years. My skin looks leathery. I have been told this and the gruffness in my voice are due to my smoking. If I should quit (and I intend to), are these conditions reversible?*

It is unlikely your skin will improve or the gravelly quality of your voice will change much if you quit smoking. However, your quitting will put a stop to further damage to these organs. Likewise the damage to your blood vessels will stop. You may find some gradual improvement in coronary artery (heart) circulation and possibly a lowering of your blood pressure.

Some techniques of sanding and abrasion may help to remove some of the wrinkles in your skin, but the leathery texture will remain. If your voice has become hoarse, you should have your throat examined by a specialist to rule out cancer.

- *Certain books are now claiming estrogen will make us look younger. Is this really possible?*

Some physicians as well as their patients have thought that estrogen exerted a "slowing" effect upon the development of wrinkles. Studies strongly suggest a beneficial effect upon the collagen within the skin when you take estrogen. This could account for a decrease in wrinkling or aging of your skin when you take the hormone.

Certainly more research is necessary in this area. But it will be interesting to see if this claim of slower aging of your skin can be proved in research studies.

- *What causes my skin to age so much after menopause?*

Fatty tissue all over your body begins to thin out and disappear in some areas. You may have noticed a decrease in the size of your breasts. When the fatty tissue disappears from beneath your skin, the skin wrinkles. These changes occur more rapidly or more slowly in different individuals. It may have something to do with the rate at which estrogen is lost.

There is some evidence to show collagen in the skin is maintained by estrogen. This may account for a decreased wrinkling when you take ERT.

- *What can I do about the coarse hair that has started growing on my face since the onset of menopausal symptoms?*

First of all, consult with a trichologist about electrolysis to remove the coarse hairs, especially if they are not too numerous.

It has been shown that Aldactone® (spironalactone) works to prevent coarse dark hair. It blocks the receptors on the hair follicles that are sensitive to testosterone (beard area of face, chest and abdomen, but not hair on head, pubic area or under arms).

Dr. Leon Speroff in the third edition of *Clinical Gynecologic Endo-crinology & Infertility*, states "The response is relatively slow and a maximal effect can be demonstrated only after 6 months of treatment.

- *In addition to taking estrogen, what can I do to keep my skin healthy?*

Here are a few suggestions to help keep your skin healthy in addition to estrogen:

1. Avoid the sun and use a sun screen. Although skin cancer is usually detected early and cured, the number of new cases is rising rapidly each year. Sometimes the treatment required can have deforming or even mutilating results. Stay away from tanning spas.

2. Stop smoking if you want to avoid the leathery, aged-appearing skin so typical of heavy smokers.

3. Avoid too-generous use of soap. A cream may be better for cleansing and for protection against drying.

4. Perfumed lotions often contain alcohol which dries your skin. Oil-base cosmetics may be preferable.

5. Moisturizers do help after a bath, certainly in the place of a drying lotion.

6. Some studies have demonstrated vitamin C may increase the amount of collagen in your skin, which could in turn slow down wrinkling. More studies should be conducted to confirm this report.

- *Will female hormones help soften my skin and improve the texture of my hair? I am having difficulty coping with the evidence of aging I see in the mirror each day.*

Certainly the female sex hormone, estrogen, does not do any harm in this regard. There is an obvious loss of texture and softness when this hormone is no longer being produced in the body. We have never been able to prove estrogen will actually soften your skin or improve the texture of your hair. But many

๛   ๛   ๛

A good way to look younger is avoid slumping. Buy a bra that will support your breasts well. Good posture along with breast and body support can help give your body the contour you desire.

women claim it has done just that for them!

Menopause can and should be a marvelous time for you. For the first time in your life, in many instances, you are completely free from the worry of pregnancy. By this time your children have probably moved away or been married. It is a time when you can begin to allow space for yourself, space in which to enlarge your educational, physical and vocational horizons.

Decide within yourself that this part of your life will be richer and even more rewarding than all that has gone before.

- *Does estrogen really relieve rheumatoid arthritis?*

Some studies by a group of endocrinologists in Holland indicate a reduced frequency of rheumatoid arthritis with the use of oral contraceptives.

When these researchers were studying the postmenopausal onset of rheumatoid arthritis in *non*-contraceptive users, they found an 80-percent reduction of rheumatoid-arthritis incidence among users of substitution hormones (estrogen-replacement therapy). These studies suggest ERT may be beneficial to those suffering from rheumatoid arthritis.

- *Will estrogen actually help women live longer?*

ERT has been shown to reduce the risk of heart attacks and strokes. It has also been shown to slow down and even halt the progress of osteoporosis. When you consider over 30,000 women die each year due to complications of osteoporotic fractures, estrogen does make women live longer.

A study at the University of Southern California Comprehensive Cancer Center in Los Angeles was carried out on 7,610 women in a retirement community in which there were 435 deaths. This study revealed a 16-percent lower mortality rate among ERT users than in those who were not taking estrogen. Most of this improved mortality was due to fewer acute myocardial infarctions (heart attacks) in women using estrogen.

Another study by the National Institutes of Health published in the Journal of the American Medical Association in 1983, covered 2,269 women between the ages of 40 and 69 during a period of 5.6 years. The death rate among women who took estrogen after menopause was only one-third as high as those who did not.

Among women who underwent a surgical menopause due to

removal of their ovaries before menopause, the death rate of those placed on estrogen was 10 times lower than those who did not take estrogen.

The answer seems to be an obvious *Yes!* Estrogen does help women live longer.

- *Can I take generic estrogens?*

No! It is very important not to let your pharmacist substitute generic estrogen. Generic estrogen can vary in dosage as much as 25 to 40% compared to the brand-name estrogens. This variation may result in a return of symptoms which were previously well controlled with the brand-name estrogen.

16

Osteoporosis & Menopause

Osteoporosis literally means your bones are too porous. Because they have lost some of their calcium, they fracture easily. To make good concrete, you must have sufficient cement in the mixture. Less than sufficient cement (such as too little calcium in your bones) will produce concrete that will crack. Likewise, bones that contain too little calcium also crack easily.

Osteoporosis is a preventable disease.

- *What causes osteoporosis?*

It is normal and common for your bones to become more porous and lose some of their calcium as you get older. Part of this is because you exercise less. Some of it may be due to a diet in which you drink less milk or simply consume too little calcium. But most osteoporosis is due to a loss of estrogen (female sex hormone) from your body, especially after menopause. Too little estrogen causes you to lose calcium from your bones.

- *What are some other common causes of osteoporosis besides loss of estrogen?*

Certain diseases (diabetes, chronic lung disease, etc.), medications (cortisone, lasix, heparin, etc.), heredity (fair skin, small frame, Caucasian, oriental), family history (hip fractures, dowager humps), nutritional factors (calcium deficiency, excessive protein intake, vitamins A, D and C, magnesium, caffeine, alcohol and smoking), lifestyle (immobilization, lack of exercise, prolonged bed rest), and hormonal deficiency during the reproductive years (excess exercise, anorexia, etc.) can all contribute or cause loss of bone mass.[1]

1 Diczfalusy, E. "Menopause, Developing Countries and The 21st Century." *Menopause.* Yearbook Medical Publishers. 1987. 1-19.

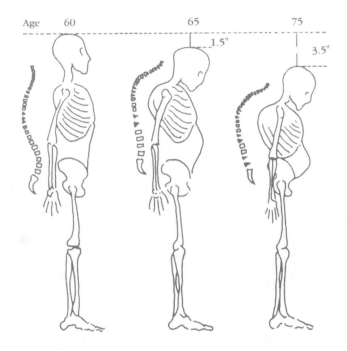

Age   60   65   75

Skeletal changes in progressing osteoporosis, called vertebral crush fracture syndrome. Progressive loss of height and increasing deformity occur as more and more vertebral bodies are compressed. Drawing courtesy of Wyeth/Ayerst Laboratories.

Certain other conditions, especially some cancers, cause osteoporosis, but these are unrelated to menopause.

- *What are the symptoms of osteoporosis? Why is osteoporosis harmful?*

For many years of its existence in a patient, osteoporosis is a silent disease. But eventually it begins to show its devastating effect. You may become aware of a backache. But the first obvious change may be a decrease in your height or even a fracture. Perhaps you have noticed how people become "bent over with age." You don't realize it, but you may be considerably shorter now than you were in your youth.

You may or may not have noticed how cautious you are becoming when sidewalks are icy or when you go up or down stairs. Possibly you know several menopausal women who have suffered from a broken hip or a broken wrist. How many menopausal women complain of what they call *lumbago*, which to them

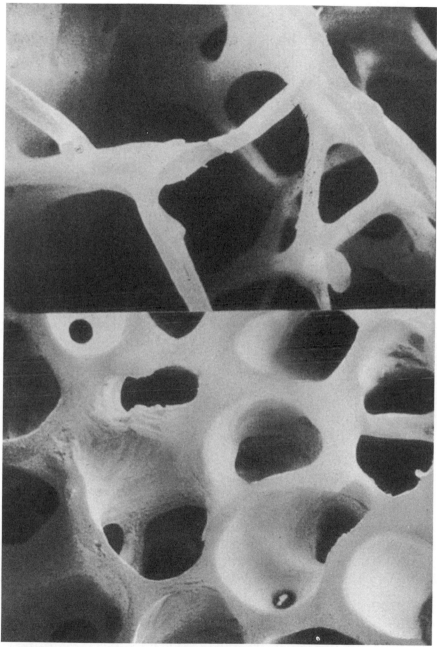

Comparison of osteoporotic bone structure above with normal bone below. These electron-microscope photos (extreme magnification!) clearly show how the bone is weakened as the structure loses bone mass through calcium loss. These photos are from a research article by Dempster, Shane and Lindsay (1986).

means backache?

Most of these symptoms are due to osteoporosis. As your bones become more porous, they lose calcium, become brittle and are more prone to fracture. One of the greatest fears of older people is falling and breaking a hip, which means a trip to the hospital.

When osteoporosis develops in your vertebrae, they also become subject to easy fracture. Because your vertebrae must support the weight of your body, they require a lot of calcium to give them strength in their framework. When calcium is lost, these vertebrae begin to collapse under your weight and you suffer what we call *compression fractures.*

Compression fractures of your vertebrae produce not only backache but also a loss of height. Your back begins to arch forward and shorten as the vertebrae collapse under the weight of your body. You may lose from 3 to 8 inches in height. The arching of your upper back is known as *dowager's hump.* It causes you to lean forward and become stooped over as you walk or stand.

- *What actually takes place in osteoporosis?*

Bone is composed of calcium and phosphorus crystals imbedded in a soft network of protein fibers. Protein is soft and pliable and gives flexibility to this framework. Calcium is then deposited along with phosphorus, fluoride, sodium, potassium, magnesium and citrate to give strength and the necessary rigidity to your bones. The correct balance between the calcium and protein network provides rigidity plus flexibility without brittleness.

Your bone is really living tissue that is constantly being "remodeled." Everyday usage causes old bone cells to be used up and replaced by new bone cells. Normally, 10 to 30 percent of your entire skeleton is remodeled each year by this bone crew. They seem to work uncomplainingly if you supply them with sufficient calcium, a well-balanced diet and stimulation from exercise. But they must have material if you expect them to work.

- *When does osteoporosis begin?*

Bones grow in length and width during childhood and adolescence. By age 18, 90 to 95 percent of bone mass has been formed. The bone-building process is fairly complete by age 25, when a modeling-remodeling process begins. For most people bone mass is fairly stable from 25 until 35 when it begins to decline gradually.

With the onset of menopause and the loss of estrogen, the demin-eralization process accelerates, causing about 5-percent[2] bone-mass loss per year for 5 years. It decreases to 1-percent loss per year thereafter. During the 20-year period after menopause, you may lose between 25 and 50 percent of your total skeletal mass.

Remember you may have been losing mass ever since age 35. Some women lose this bone mass faster than others. Thirty-per-cent loss of bone mass is the critical point at which your bones begin to fracture easily. Unfortunately you have no way of know-ing you have osteoporosis until you begin to have fractures, lose height or become stooped.

- *Do men also develop osteoporosis?*

Yes, men do develop osteoporosis. But after menopause, women lose bone mass about 6 times as fast as men until the age of 65, after which bone-loss rate slows in both sexes.

- *How common is osteoporosis?*

It is estimated 25 to 50 percent of post-menopausal women now have osteoporosis or will eventually develop osteoporosis. About 20 percent, or 1 in 5 women, have *severe* osteoporosis.

- *Why are women more likely to develop osteoporosis than men?*

Men develop osteoporosis in fewer numbers than women be-cause men are generally more muscular, weigh more (have greater bone mass) and consume more calcium. They are more likely to do heavy work or exercise more intensely. Even teenage boys have heavier and denser bones than girls. Bones respond to what is demanded of them. The more they must support in either work or exercise, the heavier and stronger they become.

Perhaps the principal reason men have less osteoporosis is they do not suffer the sudden loss of hormones women do with the loss of ovarian function during menopause.

- *Are certain women more likely to develop osteoporosis?*

For some reasons we don't understand, fair-skinned women from Northern Europe, Britain, Japan and China are the most prone to osteoporosis. Heredity plays some role in that if your mother or grandmother had osteoporosis, you have a greater

2 Stevenson, J.C. "Pathogenesis, Prevention and Treatment of Osteoporosis." *Obstetrics and Gynecology.* 1990. 75:36S–41S.

chance of developing it. Likewise, women who have breast-fed their infants, those who are allergic to milk and milk products and small-boned women seem more prone to develop osteoporosis.

The following are risk factors for developing osteoporosis:

White or Oriental
Fair complexion
Slender or slight build, low muscle mass, low bone mass
Family history of osteoporosis
Has a gastrectomy (removal of part or all of the stomach)
Takes steroids
Has certain diseases or treatment that affect calcium absorption, i.e., parathyroid disease
Sedentary, doesn't exercise or is immobilized
Smoker
Consumes alcohol (any amount contributes—the greater the amount the greater the loss)
High-protein or high-fiber diet
Drinks or takes caffeine (any amount contributes—the greater the amount the greater the loss)
Deficient diet (anorexia, marathoner, ballet dancer-dieter)
No children
Low calcium intake, especially during teens
Premature menopause because of removal of ovaries
Menopause

Elderly women: All of the above, plus history of previous fractures, tendency to fall, reduced mobility and unsafe environment.

Women who are at special risk for osteoporosis, regardless of the cause, should be treated with calcium, estrogen and an exercise program.

- *Does osteoporosis have any other effects upon women besides causing fractures?*

No one likes to become bent over. It is even worse when someone else notices before you do. Or when you suddenly notice in the mirror that you are not standing as erect as you normally do. You may notice your clothes don't fit quite as well as they used to. Or you may have chronic backache.

You may be aware your legs and your arms seem extra long in proportion to your body. You may feel less sure-footed than usual and begin to take shorter steps than you used to. When you come to stairs or curbs, you hesitate to avoid stumbling. Unless you are aware of what is happening, osteoporosis can erode your confidence and your self-esteem.

- *Why does osteoporosis affect the vertebrae in my neck more than elsewhere?*

It probably affects all of your vertebrae, causing them to fracture as the round, body-portion of the vertebrae is crushed. The deformity may be more noticeable in your neck because the curvature is more visible. Backache may be more common in your lower back where the weight-stress is greater.

- *Are there any laboratory tests to screen for osteoporosis?*

In uncomplicated cases of osteoporosis, laboratory blood testing may be helpful in identifying those who are developing osteoporosis. Two tests are especially useful to identify those who are rapidly losing calcium from their bones.

1. An elevated fasting urinary hydroxyproline/creatinine ratio (greater than 0.012).

2. An elevated fasting urinary calcium/creatinine ratio (greater than 0.16).

These tests suggest rapid bone turnover in your body. However, they are non-specific. There appears to be substantial overlap in the results between normal and osteoporotic groups of women.

- *How do I know if I am developing osteoporosis?*

Unfortunately, conventional X-rays do not show osteoporosis until about 35 percent of your bone mass has been lost. However, some newer, more-sophisticated methods are encouraging. Laboratories and clinics are springing up all over the U.S. in which serious and improved methods are being developed to detect and treat osteoporosis. Your doctor or your local hospital can direct you to these clinics. Many of these osteoporosis centers are sponsored by hospitals.

In general, bone-mass measurement for screening purposes is still a matter of considerable controversy. An article by F. M. Hall in the *New England Journal of Medicine* (1987) suggests we use risk factors to determine who should be treated.

- *Is osteoporosis painful? In other words, can I tell by pain when I am developing osteoporosis?*

  No. Remember bone loss is gradual and insidious for many years. Symptoms may not appear until enough bone mass has been lost to produce hair-line fractures that cause backache, fractures or deformity of your back. Osteoporosis has been compared to glaucoma and diabetes, in which the loss can be measured (but perhaps not *felt* by the victim) long before the more obvious blindness and/or vascular changes become apparent.

- *Are there any tests that will show I am developing osteoporosis?*

  Doctors Recker, Saville and Heaney (1978) used photon absorptiometry, osteodensitometry, and cortical-thickness measurements to indicate the extent of osteoporosis. They demonstrated that estrogens protect women from bone loss following a spontaneous (natural as opposed to surgical) menopause.

  Two other doctors, Lindsay and Aitken (1984), proved that estrogen would protect women from bone loss after they had their ovaries removed. Both studies confirmed a substantial loss of bone mass (osteoporosis) in menopausal women when they were given only a placebo (fake pill) in the place of estrogen. These women were research subjects. They were willing individuals who knew they might not be getting estrogen.

  A 24-hour test on urine gives us a clue as to bone-mass loss. If the calcium/creatinine ratio shows any change greater than 0.16, it indicates a higher-than-normal loss of calcium through the kidneys. Another test is the hydroxyproline/creatinine ratio which, if greater than 0.12, shows excessive bone-mass loss.

  CT (computer tomography) scanning may detect bone-mass loss, but it is expensive and exposes you to X-ray. More and better methods are being developed to detect osteoporosis earlier and more accurately so it can be treated and its ravages prevented.

- *There is much talk about a CAT scan to evaluate osteoporosis. How practical is this, how expensive and how necessary?*

  When used to evaluate osteoporosis, a CAT scan is similar to

*In additon to estrogen (ERT), you will need calcium,
a nutritious diet and a regular exercise program the rest
of your life to protect against osteoporosis.*

serial X-rays that are pieced together by computer to give a picture of the entire bony structure. It will give us a picture of the density of the bone and tell how severe the osteoporosis is.

Just as a mammogram at age 35 gives us a baseline picture of the breast on which any subsequent changes can be detected, a CAT scan of the bones can give us a baseline on which to judge any changes in ensuing years.

Cost varies in different parts of the country and insurance companies will not reimburse for this test. It is not something you have done repeatedly. But if there is symptomatic evidence of osteoporosis, the CAT scan can tell how severe the problem is and how fast it is progressing.

To date there is no other safe, inexpensive, reliable test for mass screening for osteoporosis.

• *I recently read that smoking causes earlier menopause and increases the risk of osteoporosis. Is this true?*

Several studies have shown women who smoke have an earlier menopause (2 years earlier) and have lower estrogen levels.[3] Both factors increase your risk of developing osteoporosis earlier. It has also been observed that smokers require higher doses of estrogen than non-smokers to achieve comparable therapeutic effects (relief from unpleasant symptoms of menopause).

• *Is there anything I might do to prevent osteoporosis?*

Prevention of osteoporosis should begin in childhood while the bone-building process is ongoing by having a nutritionally balanced diet, 1200 milligrams of calcium each day (4 glasses of milk) and developing a consistent exercise program. During the reproductive years women should maintain a good diet, exercise regularly, get 1000mg of calcium daily and refrain from smoking, alcohol, high-protein diets, excesses in caffeine, vitamins A, D and C, and minerals which may limit development of bone mass.

The second step of prevention is to take estrogen at menopause when rapid bone loss would normally begin.

The menopausal woman must also maintain a good diet (lowfat), exercise regularly, take 1200-1600mg of calcium per day in her diet, and refrain from smoking, alcohol and caffeine, etc. that

3 Gold, E.B. "Smoking and the Menopause." *Menopause Management.* Nov. 1990. III: 3:9-11.

would decrease her bone mass.

- *What kind of exercise do you recommend to prevent osteoporosis?*

When the astronauts returned to earth after their prolonged stay in space, their physicians noticed a definite loss of bone mass. Even with such a relatively short time in space, there was still a measurable reduction. The only explanation was the lack of exercise and lack of bone stress due to zero gravity. Gravity, muscle pull and exercise all combine to maintain bone mass and bone integrity.

There wasn't much the scientists could do about the lack of gravity, but they devised special stress exercises all astronauts must undertake while in space. Likewise, your bones respond to the stress and muscle pull placed upon them. Outdoor exercise gives an additional advantage. The vitamin D in sunshine helps to metabolize calcium (helps it become absorbed into your body).

If you are experiencing menopause and have never exercised, it would be foolish to begin with an intensive program. First of all, check with your doctor to see if there is any reason you shouldn't exercise or if there are certain exercises you shouldn't do. Check page 119 to find more details on exercise during menopause.

Keep in mind most people can walk and walking is a valuable exercise. Don't feel you need to jog or run immediately. Many women are frightened away from exercise because they are so out of shape to begin with. You may also have to begin with non-weight-bearing exercises (bicycling, swimming) and very gradually work into upright, weight-bearing exertion.

- *Is there a special diet to prevent osteoporosis or at least prevent it from worsening?*

Women experiencing menopause often feel they no longer need milk. They may shy away from dairy products, because they do not want to gain weight. Contrary to common opinion, you still need milk and calcium. Menopausal bone loss results from estrogen deficiency. Calcium intake alone has little effect in preventing osteoporosis.

Many women and men as they grow older develop a lactose intolerance so calcium supplements may be preferable to milk. You can find reduced-lactose milk in some areas. Sweet-acidophilus lowfat milk can also be consumed by some people who are badly affected by regular milk.

If you want to reduce calories, try 1-percent milk or even skim milk—sometimes called *nonfat*—and ice milk or nonfat frozen yogurt instead of the creamier and richer ice cream. The United States RDA (recommended daily allowance) is 800 milligrams of calcium per day for an adult. This is the minimum necessary to maintain bone mass. Many doctors and nutritionists recommend women take more calcium than quoted by the RDA. For example. it is believed that teenagers, pregnant and nursing mothers need 1,200mg of calcium each day. They recommend 1,000 milligrams per day for premenopausal women and 1,500 milligrams per day for postmenopausal women and elderly men. If for some reason you don't drink milk, take calcium tablets.

Calcium tablets come in various forms: calcium carbonate, calcium citrate, calcium gluconate, calcium lactate and calcium phosphate. Calcium carbonate is supplied under multiple trade names. It seems to be better absorbed than the others and contains 40-percent elemental calcium, considerably more than the other compounds. RDA can be met by taking only two medium-size 600-milligram tablets of calcium carbonate daily. Other calcium compounds may require anywhere from 9 to 24 tablets a day to meet your RDA requirements.

Look for the word "elemental" as it tells you how much actual calcium is in each tablet. This is true for any brand of calcium you are considering.

When you think of calcium, you naturally think of dairy products such as milk and cheese. There are also other good sources of calcium such as leafy green vegetables, salmon and raw oysters.

Because too much calcium can increase the risk of kidney stones, follow your doctor's instructions. It is true certain individuals are more likely to develop kidney stones. This is one more reason you should check with your doctor as to your own special optimum dose. We encourage women to drink 8 glasses of water per day while taking calcium supplements.

The accompanying charts show foods and list their caloric content and the amount of calcium they contain. The charts start on page 239.

The charts start on page 239.

≥&   ≥&   ≥&

Menopausal bone loss results from estrogen deficiency. Calcium intake alone has little effect in preventing osteoporosis.

- *Do certain foods increase my calcium loss? Recent magazine articles have caused me to worry about this.*

Some reliable studies have indicated excessive amounts of both protein and fat in your diet will increase the excretion of calcium from your body. Admittedly it is difficult to know just how much protein or fat is "excessive."

A 1980 report by Dr. T.G. Skillman claimed soft drinks (both diet and regular), coffee, alcohol and cigarettes all cause excessive calcium loss from the body. Many others agree.

Excessive amounts of fiber, vitamins A, C, D and some minerals may interfere with absorption of calcium from your intestinal tract.

- *I am already developing some humping in my back despite my efforts to improve my posture. I am also overweight and have been looking at various diets. Should certain diets be avoided when osteoporosis is developing?*

The so-called low-calorie, high-protein diets may produce acidosis over the long haul, which in turn causes you to lose more calcium through your kidneys. Such diets will aggravate your osteoporosis.

Other diets that exclude calcium might also be harmful. The same could be said for consuming too much caffeine, because this could also produce some acidosis. The *National Women's Health Report* (1986) stated, "Caffeine acts to disrupt the kidneys' ability to reabsorb calcium." The best way to lose weight is to combine lowfat eating with a sensible exercise program.

- *Will estrogen prevent actual fractures, the loss of height and the deformity (humping of my back) that come with osteoporosis?*

Estrogen can stop progression of the disease of osteoporosis, but it will not reverse any changes that have already occurred. For instance, if you have already developed some curvature of your spine due to compression fractures of your vertebrae, estrogen will not help to straighten your spine.

If you are having backache due to these vertebral-compression fractures, you should not expect these backaches to be completely relieved. What you can expect is future fractures or a progression of the disease can be prevented or slowed down.

A study by Henneman and Wallach as early as 1957 showed

estrogen will prevent osteoporosis from progressing. The women they tested had already lost up to 5 inches in height due to osteoporosis. When followed for 25 years, they found the "shrinking" was halted when the estrogen was begun.

Dr. Lila Nachtigall (1979) of New York University School of Medicine conducted a 10-year study in which she demonstrated that estrogen-replacement therapy begun within 3 years after menopause actually *increased* a woman's bone mass. She also showed estrogen started after 3 years past menopause will stop bone loss, but will not increase bone mass.

- *What effect do estrogens have on osteoporosis?*

Women lose only an insignificant amount of calcium from their bones as long as they are having menstrual periods. But when estrogen production goes down and menopause begins, there is a rapid increase in calcium loss. It is interesting that bone-mass loss varies according to estrogen rather than age. This means women who menstruate into their 50s still do not suffer increased calcium loss until their periods stop.

Dr. Robert Lindsay (1984) conducted a 9-year, double-blind study in Scotland. His study showed women on estrogen-replacement therapy did not lose height, whereas those who were not on estrogen did. In 1983, the Council on Scientific Affairs of the American Medical Association published a statement concluding estrogen effectively prevents osteoporosis.

In 1984, the advisory panel of the United States Government's National Institutes of Health gave a strong endorsement to the use of estrogen for the prevention of osteoporosis. In 1986 the FDA approved estrogen for the treatment and prevention of osteoporosis.

The evidence is overwhelming. Dr. Robert Lindsay put it well when he said, "Estrogens are the single most potent pharmacological factor to reduce the loss of bone mass and to protect a woman against osteoporosis."

Hip fractures are serious accidents for older women. In a study by Burch, Bird and Vaughn of 14,318 patient years of estrogen use by women who had had hysterectomies (including removal of their ovaries), there were no hip fractures and a significant reduction in the number of wrist fractures. Countless other studies have confirmed these findings. A patient year is one patient using estrogen for one year.

- *I have heard estrogen will increase my chance of developing cancer in my uterus. Is this true?*

First of all, let us say that women who have had a hysterectomy can take estrogen without any worry in this regard. If you still have your uterus, there is a chance that estrogen, if taken alone, can increase your chance of developing cancer of the lining of your uterus. It is true your risk increases from about 0.7 cases per 1,000 to about 3 per 1,000.

Because endometrial cancer causes bleeding, this type of cancer is usually discovered early and the 5-year cure rate is about 95 percent. But even more important than the high cure rate is the fact there is practically no danger of increased cancer risk if you take progestogen along with estrogen.

Progestogen can be taken as medroxyprogesterone (Provera®) 10mgm, or norethindrome acetate (Norlutate®) 5mgm for 12 to 13 days each month along with estrogen to protect you against any increased risk of cancer.

- *Will estrogens increase my risk of breast cancer?*

Multiple studies done over the last 30 years have not shown estrogen to cause breast cancer. There seem to be multiple factors that interplay to put women at risk for developing breast cancer. Diet and heredity have also been suggested. Researchers are now looking at chromosomes 10 and 13 for possible clues to heredity.[4]

- *How much estrogen should I take?*

The dose needed to relieve menopausal symptoms may vary with each patient, but the dose known to prevent osteoporosis is 0.625 milligrams per day of conjugated estrogen.

- *Will the estrogen I take after I am through menopause cause me to start having menstrual periods again?*

About 70 percent of our patients on the 0.625-milligram dose of conjugated estrogen (or 0.05mg/day skin patch) combined with 12 to 13 days of Provera® have bleeding each month. Many stop bleeding after 1 to 2 years or have only a light period. Check with your doctor carefully so dosages can be adjusted to your needs,

---

4 Nachtigall, L.E. "Estrogen Replacement Therapy and Breast Cancer." *Current Perspective on Managing the Premenopausal and Postmenopausal Patient.* Dec. 8, 1990. New York University Postgraduate Medical School Conference. Dallas, TX.

giving you only the lowest dosage you require.

- *Will I have to take hormones indefinitely to avoid osteoporosis?*

  Yes. Based on recent research, your chances of developing osteoporosis are decreased by 50 to 60 percent if you have been taking estrogen for at least 6 years. Estrogens can be effective until at least the age of 80 (Gambrell 1985), and we now feel they will be protective throughout your lifetime. In fact, many doctors advise women in their 80s to continue estrogen-replacement therapy to protect them from bone-mass loss.

- *Are there any other precautions I should take while on estrogen and progestogen?*

  1. Report any bleeding other than at the expected time (when your doctor told you to expect it, based upon your estrogen progestogen schedule). All intermenstrual spotting is considered abnormal until its cause is determined by your doctor.

  2. Continue to make regular annual visits to your doctor to have a Pap smear, a pelvic and rectal exam and a breast exam, including a mammogram if over 50. Your doctor may want to give you a complete physical examination.

  3. An annual lipid profile which evaluates the good and bad cholesterol components in your blood is also a good idea, especially if you have a family history of cardiovascular disease. If this lipid profile is abnormal, a strict lowfat diet (limited saturated fats and high cholesterol foods) may be necessary.

  4. If any unpleasant symptoms develop, discuss them with your doctor so dosages or types of medication can be adjusted or changed. Don't just stop taking the medications on your own.

- *I have heard 40 to 50 percent of women will never develop osteoporosis, especially if they are fairly plump or black and have a late menopause. I fit this picture perfectly. There is no history of heart attacks or stroke in my family. Why should I take ERT?*

  You may well be the exception, but the general rule is still valid. Nearly all women benefit from estrogen-replacement therapy after menopause. Your skin, hair, vaginal mucous membranes, libido and several other systems may also benefit from ERT.

- *I have severe osteoporosis, have lost about 6 inches in height, and have a deforming curvature of my back. Is there any hope some of this bone can be rebuilt by taking estrogen and calcium?*

According to recent studies by Dr. Lila Nachtigall (1987), who has studied osteoporosis for over 15 years, there is encouraging information. When estrogen is started during the first 3 years after menopause, bone mass appears to be added. Dr. Edward Lufkin from Mayo Clinic reported on studies at Mayo Clinic showing that women over 70 benefit from ERT in the form of the estrogen patch. These studies showed that estrogens are safe and effective in the treatment of osteoporosis. Women in the studies showed increased bone-mineral content in the lumbar spine and hip with reduced vertebral-fracture rate.[5]

- *What about taking calcium? Is there an age limit, or do I need to take calcium tablets for the rest of my life so I will not develop osteoporosis?*

If you take sufficient calcium in your diet, if you are a heavy consumer of milk, cheese and other dairy products, you might not have to take calcium supplements at all. Most menopausal women drink coffee or tea rather than milk. In general, most menopausal women need to take supplemental calcium.

Prior to menopause you should have 1,000 milligrams of calcium in your daily diet. There are 3 special periods in your life in which 1,200 milligrams of dietary calcium are recommended: during teenage years, pregnancy and during lactation (nursing).

Once you begin menopause, because of decreased absorption in your intestinal tract, *increase* your calcium intake to 1,200-1,600 milligrams a day. If your diet can't supply enough calcium, take calcium tablets.

Although calcium loss decreases after age 65, it does continue. Most physicians feel you should continue to take calcium supplements for the rest of your life.

The exception to this advice is those women who have a tendency to form kidney stones. If you have this problem, seek the advice of your physician.

5 Lufkin, E.G. "Estrogen Efficacy and Side Effect in the Prevention and Treatment of Osteoporosis." *Current Perspective on Managing the Premenopausal and Postmenopausal Woman.* Dec. 8, 1990. New York University Postgraduate Medical School. Dallas, TX.

- *I have had calcium kidney stones in the past. Now I'm in menopause and need calcium to prevent osteoporosis. What should I do?*

First of all, check with your doctor. He may feel the risk of kidney stones is greater than the risk of osteoporosis. If you take calcium, you may find calcium citrate is less likely to form kidney stones.

Increase your fluid intake to at least 8 or 10 glasses of water per day. Your doctor may give you a thiazide diuretic to decrease your urinary calcium loss. After you have been evaluated, your doctor will advise the best program of treatment for you.

In summary, the best treatment for osteoporosis in menopausal women is to take estrogen in the dose your doctor feels best for you. You will probably need 1,200 to 1,600 milligrams of calcium daily along with a sensible exercise program to round out your treatment and prevent osteoporosis.

Osteoporosis is preventable and treatable!

- *Is there any special brand of calcium I should take?*

The average menopausal woman should take about 1,200 to 1,600 milligrams of elemental calcium daily. Of the various calcium compounds the best tolerated seems to be calcium carbonate, but individual tastes vary when it comes to the brand. It is possible you will tolerate one brand better than another.

If you have side effects, check with your pharmacist and have him give you a different brand.

- *Should every postmenopausal woman take calcium supplements?*

Very few women eat enough calcium-containing foods to supply their needs. You need at least 1,200mg daily if you take estrogen and 1,600mg daily if you do not take estrogen. So the answer is yes, you do need supplemental calcium.

You especially need supplemental calcium if you are vegetarian, if you eat a high-fiber diet (fiber causes less absorption of calcium) and if you take antacids. Don't take all your calcium with antacids or iron medication. It is best to take them at bedtime so calcium does not compete with food or medications for absorption.

- *Many in my family have osteoporosis. I have heard fluoride and vitamin D, if given along with calcium, will give even better results than calcium alone. Is this true?*

At the Mayo Clinic, Dr. L. Rigg has had an ongoing study for over 20 years in which he has evaluated various combinations of therapy for osteoporosis. Naturally those patients on calcium fared better than those who took no calcium. The group that took calcium plus fluoride had only 61 percent as many fractures as those on calcium alone.

The best results were in those women treated with ERT, calcium and fluoride. The addition of vitamin D caused some women to develop too much calcium in their blood, and it had to be discontinued. In the United States we have plenty of sunlight along with many foods that have been fortified with vitamin D, so we shouldn't have to take a vitamin D supplement.

The Mayo Clinic Group did not recommend fluoride because the bone that was laid down appeared to be abnormal and more brittle. Large doses of fluoride used in this study also caused some intestinal upset along with rheumatic-type joint pains.

- *Will fluoride help prevent fractures due to osteoporosis?*

Some recent studies from both Finland and Yugoslavia indicate fluoride does have some protective effect against fractures in women who have osteoporosis. But no one knows what the fluoride dosage is that will make a stronger, denser bone that is not abnormal in formation or brittle. However, these women should still take estrogen to prevent further progression of the osteoporotic process.

- *I have read fair-skinned, small-boned, smoking, drinking women with ancestors from Northern Europe who have an early menopause are more likely to develop osteoporosis. I fit none of these descriptions. Does that mean I don't have to worry about osteoporosis?*

Those women are more prone to develop osteoporosis. The fact that only 50 percent or fewer women develop severe osteoporosis does not mean you should not take precautions to avoid it. Add to this the fact ERT (estrogen-replacement therapy) may help you live longer, protect you against cardiovascular disease, stall some of the skin changes, bladder changes, vaginal-tissue changes and generally make you feel better. You may consider taking it.

If you live long enough, you will lose 40 percent or more of your bone mass. At least one-third of women who live to be 60 will have symptomatic osteoporosis. And 1.3 million of these women will have bone fractures, mostly fractured hips, wrists and also fractured vertebrae that cause them to hump over.

In addition to the cost, pain and inconvenience, about 30,000 women die each year due to complications of these fractures.

Another 300,000 require long-term care. This is care that may extend beyond their insurance coverage.

- *What does alcohol have to do with osteoporosis?*

Alcohol interferes with calcium absorption. In heavy drinkers, it often takes the place of food, including calcium-containing foods.

- *Does osteoporosis affect the teeth?*

In the *Archives of Internal Medicine,* 1983, there is an article by Harry W. Daniell, M.D. in which he finds a greater loss of teeth due to periodontal disease and osteoporosis in white women after menopause. We know of no other studies.

- *Is a woman ever too old to take ERT to halt progress of osteoporosis or other symptoms such as vaginal tenderness?*

No. We have treated many women in their 80s and some in their 90s. All have benefited.

- *Besides taking estrogen, are there any other things I should do to help prevent osteoporosis?*

There are two things that will help. We already know exercise will thicken and strengthen your bones. Your bones respond to the stress placed upon them. If you are exercising, your bones must handle the pull and stress the muscles place upon them. Exercise helps to prevent osteoporosis.

You may find you should take supplemental calcium, especially if you have trouble eating enough dairy products and other foods that contain calcium. Sunshine might help supply vitamin D, which also increases your absorption of calcium.

- *I have recently read about etidronate as a new treatment for osteoporosis. Is this something I should consider because I have recently been told I have osteoporosis and cannot take estrogen because of breast cancer?*

Etidronate-disodium (Didronel®) as of early 1991 had not yet been FDA-approved for the treatment of osteoporosis. Two recent studies showed that the use of etidronate increased vertebral-bone-mineral content (backbone) by 5.3 percent and the rate of new vertebral fractures (compressing or cracking) were decreased by 50 percent.[6,7] These studies are promising as they show etidronate may be an alternative form of therapy (other than estrogen or calcitonin) for treating osteoporosis.

6 Watts, N.B., et al. "Intermittent Cyclical Etidronate Treatment of Postmenopausal Osteoporosis." *New England Journal of Medicine.* 1990:323:73-9.
7 Storm, T. et al. "Effect of Intermittent Cyclical Etidronate Therapy on Bone Mass and Fracture Rates in Women with Postmenopausal Osteoporosis." *New England Journal of Medicine.* 1990. 322:1265-1271.

Calcium & Caloric Content of Foods*

Food	Amount	Ca(mg)	Calories	Food	Amount	Ca(mg)	Calories
Dairy Products				Shrimp, canned	3 oz	98	99
Milk				Soups			
Whole, 3.5%	1 cup	288	159	Canned (prepared			
Nonfat (skim)	1 cup	296	88	with water)			
Butter, stick	½ cup	23	812.5	Clam chowder	1 cup	34	81
Buttermilk	1 cup	296	88	Cream of chicken	1 cup	24	94
Cheese				Cream of			
Blue or Roquefort	1 cu in	54	64	mushroom	1 cup	41	134
Camembert	1 wedge	40	114	Minestrone	1 cup	37	105
Cheddar	1 cu in	129	68	Tuna, canned in oil,			
Cottage	12 oz	320	360	drained	3 oz	7	167
Parmesan, grated	1 tbsp	68	23	**Vegetables**			
Swiss (natural)	1 cu in	139	56				
Swiss (processed)	1 cu in	159	64	Asparagus, green	1 cup	37	36
American	1 cu in	122	65	Beans			
Cream				Lima	1 cup	80	189
Half-and-half	1 tbsp	16	20	Red kidney	1 cup	74	218
Light	1 tbsp	15	32	Snap (green or			
Sour	1 tbsp	12	22	yellow)	1 cup	72	31
Custard, baked	1 cup	297	305	Beets	1 cup	29	58
Ice cream	1 cup	194	257	Broccoli, cooked	1 stalk	158	47
Ice milk				Brussels sprouts	1 cup	50	56
Hardened	1 cup	204	199	Cabbage			
Soft-serve	1 cup	273	266	Raw	1 cup	39	20
Margarine, stick	½ cup	23	816	Cooked	1 cup	64	29
Pudding				Red, raw, coarsely			
Chocolate	1 cup	250	385	shredded	1 cup	29	22
Vanilla	1 cup	298	283	Carrots	1 cup	45	48
Yogurt				Cashew nuts	1 cup	53	785
made from whole				Cauliflower, cooked	1 cup	25	28
milk	1 cup	272	152	Celery, pieces	1 cup	39	20
made from				Collards, cooked	1 cup	289	51
partially				Mustard greens,			
skimmed milk	1 cup	294	123	cooked	1 cup	193	32
Meat, Poultry & Seafood				Onions			
				Raw	1 onion	30	44
Beef, lean only	2½ oz	10	153	Cooked	1 cup	50	61
Chicken breast, fried	2½ oz	9	160	Parsnips, cooked	1 cup	70	102
Eggs				Peanuts, roasted	1 cup	107	838
Whole	1 egg	27	82	Peas, green	1 cup	44	114
Yolk of egg	1 yolk	24	59	Pumpkin, canned	1 cup	57	81
Scrambled with				Sauerkraut, canned	1 cup	85	42
milk and fat	1 egg	51	111	Spinach	1 cup	200	41
Clams	3 oz	53	65	Squash, cooked	1 cup	55	129
Crabmeat, canned	3 oz	38	91	Sweet potatoes	1 med	52	185
Haddock, breaded,				Tomatoes	1 med	24	40
fried	3 oz	34	141	Tomato catsup	1 cup	60	289
Oysters, raw	1 cup	226	158	Turnips, cooked	1 cup	54	36
Salmon, pink, canned	3 oz	167	120	Turnip greens,			
Sardines, canned in				cooked	1 cup	252	28
oil, drained	3 oz	372	174				

Food	Amount	Ca(mg)	Calories	Food	Amount	Ca(mg)	Calories
Fruits & Fruit Products				Farina, cooked	1 cup	147	105
Apricots				Muffins, enriched			
Canned in heavy				white flour	1 muffin	42	118
syrup	1 cup	28	222	Oats	1 cup	44	99
Dried, uncooked	1 cup	100	338	Oatmeal	1 cup	22	132
Avocados	1 med	26	378	Pancakes			
Blackberries, raw	1 cup	46	84	Wheat flour	1 cake	27	62
Blueberries, raw	1 cup	21	90	Plain or buttermilk	1 cake	58	61
Cantaloupes, raw,				Pie			
medium	½ melon	27	82	Butterscotch	4-in sec	98	344
Cherries, canned, red	1 cup	37	105	Custard	4-in sec	125	280
Dates, pitted	1 cup	105	488	Mince	4-in sec	38	364
Grapefruit, pink	½ med	20	50	Pecan	4-in sec	55	488
Grapefruit juice	1 cup	23	96	Pumpkin	4-in sec	166	272
Grape juice (canned				Pizza, cheese	5½ in sec	107	153
or bottled)	1 cup	28	167	Rice, cooked	1 cup	21	223
Lime juice	1 cup	22	64	Rolls			
Oranges	1 med	54	71	Frankfurter or			
Orange juice	1 cup	26	112	hamburger	1 roll	30	119
Papayas, raw	1 cup	36	73	Hard	1 roll	24	156
Peaches, dried	1 cup	77	419	Spaghetti with			
Pineapple, raw	1 cup	27	81	meatballs			
Pineapple juice,				Home recipe	1 cup	124	332
canned	1 cup	37	138	Canned	1 cup	53	258
Plums, canned	1 cup	36	114	Waffles			
Prunes, cooked	1 cup	60	253	Enriched flour	1 waffle	85	209
Prune juice, bottled	1 cup	36	197	From mix	1 waffle	179	206
Raspberries, raw	1 cup	27	70				
Rhubarb, cooked	1 cup	212	381	**Sugars & Sweets**			
Strawberries, raw	1 cup	31	55	Caramels	1 oz	42	113
Tangerines	1 med	34	39	Chocolate, milk,			
Watermelon	4-in wedge	30	111	plain	1 oz	65	147
				Fudge, plain	1 oz	22	113
Grain Products				Molasses, blackstrap	1 tbsp	137	43
Barley	1 cup	32	698	Sherbet	1 cup	31	259
Biscuits, homemade	1 biscuit	34	103	Sugar, brown	1 cup	187	821
Bran flakes with				**Nuts & Tofu**			
raisins	1 cup	28	144	Almonds	½ cup	160	425
Bread	1 slice	23	74	Pecans	½ cup	42	406
Cakes (from mixes)	1 piece	55	308	Tofu (soybean curd)	3½ oz	128	72
Cupcakes (from				Walnuts	½ cup	50	326
mixes)	1 small	43	88				
Cornmeal	1 cup	23	433				

*Calcium content derived from Krause MV, Mahan LK: *Food, nutrition and diet therapy.* Philadelphia, WB Saunders Co, 1979, p 828.

Calcium charts are from "Osteoporosis— Is it in your Future," a publication of Marion Laboratories, Inc.

17

Your Life Ahead

There was a time when women did not have to worry much about life after menopause because so few reached that age. We can almost call menopause a 20th-century phenomenon. At the turn of the century the average life expectancy was about 45 years. If you make it to menopause (average age 50) nowadays, you may expect to live for another 34 years. Some statisticians say 42 years. Just think, you have more than a third of your life ahead of you!

Life Expectancy of North-American Females After 70					
Age	Expectancy	Age	Expectancy	Age	Expectancy
70	13.9 years	76	10.3 years	81	7.8 years
71	13.3	77	9.7	82	7.3
72	12.6	78	9.2	83	6.9
73	12.0	79	8.7	84	6.5
74	11.4	80	8.2	85	6.1
75	10.8				

These years ahead are free of pregnancy, free of child-rearing, free of menstrual cramps and flow. Yet your years are now full of maturity, experience, better financial know-how and usually more security. You may have achieved a certain status in the neighborhood and community, if not in a wider circle. Menopause is not the end but the beginning—the open door to a new world in which countless opportunities offer themselves to you. So what could you possibly have questions about? Let's discuss a few of them.

- *It seems as though I have become super-conservative and super-cautious. As a result, I don't have as much fun as I did before I went through menopause. Should I be concerned?*

You have become more mature, which means you have learned from your mistakes. Naturally you are more cautious, and there is nothing wrong with that.

Youth is associated with more adventure, more recklessness and definitely more mistakes. Do you want to make all of those mistakes over again? As far as fun is concerned, we have a tendency to remember the good times and forget the bad ones. If faced with the "good old times" as they *really* were, few people would want to do more than reminisce about them.

- *How do I learn to live with increasing wrinkles, bags under my eyes that seem more prominent each morning and knuckles that are slowly getting thicker?*

One suggestion: Be thankful those wrinkles can still smile, your eyes can still see the world over the bags and you can still use your hands. Your life will be just about as good as you decide you want it to be. *You* determine what your outlook will be.

Most people love and respect wrinkles in those older than themselves. In fact, you occupy a rather honored position both in your family and in society. But no one likes to be around constantly complaining older persons, regardless of who they are.

For the most part, it is not your condition or illness you must live with but your attitude about your condition. If you can improve your attitude about yourself, you will not only improve your health, but you may improve the way others feel about you.

- *I seem to worry so much more than I ever used to, especially about my health. How can I get over this habit?*

Knowledge is one of the best cures for uncertainty, and worry is a stepchild of uncertainty. If you are worried about your health, visit your doctor for a complete check-up and eliminate the uncertainties.

Here are a few suggestions for your annual health checklist:

1. If you don't already have a good physician, find one. Find a physician with whom you can communicate and in whom you have confidence. Find one who will give you advice you will follow. Don't just look for someone to provide an examination.

2. If you smoke—quit.

3. Either stop drinking alcohol entirely or limit yourself to no more than 2 drinks at a sitting and a total of 2 drinks a day.

4. Eat a lowfat, low-salt, high-fiber diet. You do not need as many calories as you used to. Check the following weight scale to see what your normal weight should be, and lose those extra pounds. However, because muscle is denser than fat, a more-muscular person will be smaller in size than a "fatter" person, even though they are the same height and weight. Thus, your measurements, the size you wear and how your clothes fit are sometimes better guides for optimum weight.

5. Take estrogen, especially if your doctor feels you need it. Most doctors now agree nearly every woman needs estrogen to prevent osteoporosis and cardiovascular disease, as well as to treat and relieve other symptoms of menopause.

6. Take calcium and drink 8 glasses of water a day. Water helps prevent kidney stones and also prevents constipation.

7. Exercise regularly within your limits, preferably with aerobic-type exercises or sports. See Chapter 9 on Fitness & Menopause.

8. Eliminate stress as much as possible. Some things you can't change, others you can. If you can't change circumstances, maybe you can change your attitude about them.

9. Keep up your shots. This means you should have a flu shot each year, a tetanus-diptheria booster every 10 years and even a TB skin test every 10 years.

10. Have your eyes checked for glaucoma every 2 or 3 years.

11. Have your hearing checked every 5 years or more often if you find you are missing parts of conversation.

12. Have your blood pressure checked once a year. There are automatic blood-pressure machines (most are free) in your local bank and in shopping malls and other public places.

13. Buckle your seat belt before you turn on the key in your car. Learn to drive defensively.

14. Check your breasts each month after your menstrual period or by the calendar if you are beyond menopause. Have your doctor check your breasts at each annual visit.

Weights for Women 25 and Older in pounds according to height & weight, indoor clothing			
Height	Weight Small Frame	Weight Medium Frame	Weight Large Frame
4 feet 10 inches	92–98	96–107	104–119
4 feet 11 inches	94–101	98–110	106–122
5 feet	96–104	101–113	109–125
5 feet 1 inch	99–107	104–116	112–128
5 feet 2 inches	102-110	107–119	115–131
5 feet 3 inches	105–113	110–122	118–134
5 feet 4 inches	108–116	113–126	121–138
5 feet 5 inches	111–119	116–130	125–142
5 feet 6 inches	114–123	120–135	129–146
5 feet 7 inches	118–127	124–139	133–150
5 feet 8 inches	122–131	128143	137–154
5 feet 9 inches	126–135	132–147	141–158
5 feet 10 inches	130–140	136–151	145163
5 feet 11 inches	134–144	140–155	149–169
6 feet	138–148	144–159	153–173

15. Have a baseline mammogram at age 35, again at age 40, every 2 years until the age of 50 and yearly thereafter.

16. Have a pelvic and rectal exam every year.

17. Have your stool checked for occult blood (not visible to the naked eye) annually.

18. Have a proctosigmoidoscopy exam to check your rectum and lower bowel every 3 to 5 years.

19. Have a Pap smear every 1 to 3 years. If you have one every year, it gets you in for a complete exam which may turn up other problems so they can be treated early.

20. Have urine and blood tests (hematocrit, chemistry panel that includes cholesterol, sugar and other tests, which are all done from a tiny sample of blood) every few years.

21. Check with your doctor before beginning any strenuous new exercise or sport.

22. Have an electrocardiogram every 5 years.

23. Have any other tests your doctor recommends.

This seems like a long, formidable list, and you may already be

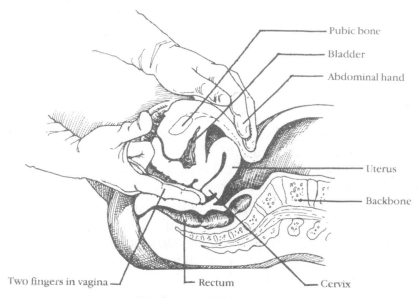

In a bimanual pelvic examination, the doctor uses pressure from above with his abdominal hand against the two fingers in the vagina to outline pelvic organs and detect abnormalities of size and contour.

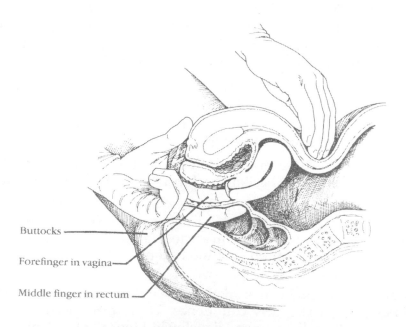

A rectovaginal pelvic examination is a pelvic exam in which your doctor can feel abnormalities in your rectum (polyps, hemorrhoids, strictures) and feel behind your uterus.

on a healthy course in your life. But all of these items become more important the older you get.

• *Why do so many postmenopausal women become fat?*

As we discussed in chapter 7, page 97, on Weight Control & Menopause, weight gain is usually not sudden but gradual. It is true that obesity is often hereditary. Some of us must battle the bulge more intensely than others. But much of the weight gain of midlife is due to a change in lifestyle rather than overeating. You are not as active as you used to be, yet you probably eat about the same as you have eaten all of your life.

Many studies have shown most women can lose weight simply by exercising regularly every day—with no change in diet. If you want a more rapid weight loss, exercise more vigorously and for a longer time. Your weight will change even faster if you make just a few changes in your diet.

Before joining an expensive spa or buying special diet-salon foods and pills, try these suggestions:

1. Avoid all sweets, pastries, desserts, soft drinks, ice cream, whipped cream and nuts.

2. Eat bread, potatoes, rice and whole grains. But leave off the extras you normally add to them, whether it be jam, honey, butter, margarine or other rich, creamy spreads.

3. Eat lots of salads. Use spices and vinegar for dressings instead of mayonnaise and other rich dressings.

4. Eat fruits and vegetables. Carrot sticks and celery sticks are excellent snacks for between meals.

5. You may have better luck with 4 or 5 small meals than with 3 large meals. Don't hesitate to skip a meal when you don't feel hungry.

6. No "seconds" at any meal. Losing weight is often the best psychotherapy there is. If you are losing pounds, you often find you lose other problems and find new energy, new drive and a new self-image.

Many women make their menopause a time of motivation with a new look and a new confidence. They seize the marvelous opportunity to discover and develop hidden talents. Menopause can be the period in your life in which long-suppressed goals can surface. You may elect to return to school for that degree or special training you would have completed in your 20s if your family hadn't come along.

Find out today where special classes for adults are offered and what you need to do to enroll in them.

If you've never played golf, take some lessons. If you've always wished you could play tennis, now you have the time. One of our patients learned to ski at age 55 and has stayed with it!

Plan for some trips you've always dreamed about but couldn't take because your family came first. Another patient of ours has taken classes to learn Spanish so she can converse as she visits Mexico.

- *So many of my friends have developed high blood pressure by the time they are 45 or 50. Is this a normal part of aging? How can I avoid it?*

Many populations isolated in such areas as South America and Polynesia have no high blood pressure at all. But when these same people migrate to our country to adopt our modern ways of living, they soon fall into the same stress patterns. The result is the development of high blood pressure.

In three nomadic tribes in northern Kenya, no single case of high blood pressure was found—and not one case of obesity was found either. About all we can say is high blood pressure does not have to be a normal part of midlife or of aging.

- *How common is high blood pressure?*

Estimates vary from 20 percent to as high as 35 percent. But we know high blood pressure is one of the most common causes of heart disease and strokes.

Here are a few suggestions to help you avoid high blood pressure and even help restore it to normal if you've already developed it:

1. Keep your weight at normal levels. If you are overweight, begin now to lose the extra pounds. Enlist your doctor's help.

2. Exercise regularly. Exercise will definitely help lower your blood pressure. Check with your doctor first to see if there are any limitations.

3. Stop smoking and limit your alcohol.

4. Leave salt out of your diet or use salt substitutes.

5. If your blood pressure is elevated, let your doctor prescribe medicine to lower it while you are working on the first four

suggestions.

6. Estrogen is thought by many to lower blood pressure. At least we know it will not elevate your blood pressure. It should be taken along with progestogen to relieve menopausal symptoms and to prevent osteoporosis.

- *It seems as though diabetes is more common during menopause. Is this true?*

It is true your body handles sugar better when you are younger and becomes less tolerant of sugar as you get older. When your body reaches the point it cannot handle all the sugar you eat, more and more of this sugar is retained by your liver. When this sugar then penetrates into the blood stream and is carried to your tissues, you may develop what we call *maturity-onset diabetes*. This type of diabetes is usually less severe, more easily controlled and less damaging than diabetes that occurs earlier in life.

Maturity-onset diabetes is definitely more common in women who are overweight or even obese. In fact, many of these women can control or even eliminate this type of diabetes by returning to a normal weight, especially in the earlier stages.

Here are a few suggestions to avoid (or improve your outlook if you already have) maturity-onset diabetes.

1. Reduce your body weight to normal.

2. Avoid overeating.

3. Eat 5 small meals, rather than 3 large meals each day.

4. Avoid sweets or sugar-sweetened foods.

5. Exercise regularly.

Although maturity-onset diabetes is not considered to be a disease of menopause, it may choose this special time in your life to show its unwanted face.

- *I know it sounds foolish, but I want to look younger. In fact, I don't care whether it's plastic surgery, hormones or what. I just want to look younger!*

Having treated thousands of women your age, we can understand what you are saying and how you feel. And yes, there are many different procedures and medicines that can help.

How you feel now and in the future will depend on how you feel about yourself.

Before you undertake plastic surgery, for instance, take a look in the mirror and decide you like the person you are looking at. Perhaps you might enjoy a new hair-do, a new type of make-up, a new outfit of clothes, a totally new look!

If you still want to get rid of the wrinkles and creases, then consider a face lift or whatever. But unless your attitude is one of self-acceptance, such procedures will not give you the satisfaction you are looking for.

Summary

Menopause and midlife bring many changes and many challenges. With a positive outlook and an aggressive approach to preventive health care, your postmenopausal years can be the *best* years of your life.

Bibliography

American Cancer Society. January/February 1987. Vol. 37, No. 1.

Avioli, L.V. "Adjunctive Modes of Therapy for Postmenopausal Osteoporosis." *Postgraduate Medicine.* Special Report, Sept. 1987:21-8.

Bachmann, C.A. et al. "Vaginal Atrophy in Postmenopausal Dyspareunia." *Female Patient.* 1984. Vol. 9:118-27.

Bachmann, C.A. et al. "Sexual Repercussions of Aging." *Contemporary OB/Gyn.* 1987. Vol. 29: 1-72.

Baker, T.C. "Oogenesis and Ovulation." *Reproduction in Mammals: Germ Cells and Fertilization.* Editors: C.R. Austin and R.V. Short. Cambridge University Press. 1978.

Baker, T.C. "Development of the Ovary and Oogeneses." *Clinical Obstetrics & Gynecology* 1976. 3:26.

Bates, G.W. "On the Nature of the Hot Flash." *Clinical Obstetrics and Gynecology.* 1981. Vol. 24:2331-241.

Beard, M.K.; Curtis, L.R. "Libido, Menopause and Estrogen Replacement Therapy." *Postgraduate Medicine.* 1989. 86:1:225-228.

Brincat, M. et al. "A Study of the Decrease of Skin Collagen Content, Skin Thickness and Bone Mass in the Postmenopausal Woman." *Abstract of Gynecology.* 1987. Vol. 70:40-5.

Brincat, M. et al. "Long-Term Effects of the Menopause and Sex Hormones on Skin Thickness." *British Journal of Obstetrics and Gynecology.* 1985. Vol. 92:256-9.

Bullock, J.L. et al. "Use of Medroxyprogesterone Acetate to Prevent Menopausal Symptoms." *Obstetrics and Gynecology.* 1975. Vol. 46, No. 2:165-8.

Bush, T.L. et al. "Estrogen Use and All Cause Mortality." *JAMA, Journal of the American Medical Association* 1983. Vol. 249:903-6.

Center for Disease Control: Cancer and Steroid Hormone Study. "Long-Term Oral Contraceptive Use and the Risk of Breast Cancer." *JAMA.* 1983. Vol. 249, No. 12:1591-1604.

Chang, R.J. and H.L. Judd. "The Ovary after Menopause." *Clinical Obstetrics and Gynecology.* March 1981. Vol. 24, No. 1.

Chetkowski, R.J. et al. "Biologic Effects of Transdermal Estradiol." *New England Journal of Medicine.* 1986. Vol. 314:1615-20.

Christiansen, C. et al. "Pathophysiological Mechanisms of Estrogen Effect on Bone Metabolism Dose-Response Relationships in Early Postmenopausal Women." *Journal of Clinical Endocrinology & Metabolism.* 1982. Vol. 55:1124-30.

Christiansen, J.J. et al. "Cigarette Smoking, Serum Estrogens and Bone Loss During Hormone Replacement Early After Menopause." *New England Journal of Medicine.* 1985. Vol. 313:973.

Colditz, C.A. et al. "Menopause and the Risk of Coronary Heart Disease in Women." *New England Journal of Medicine.* 1987. Vol. 316:1105-10.

Collins, J. et al. "Estrogen Use and Survival in Endometrial Cancer." *Lancet.* November 1980:961-4.

Coulan, C.B. "Age, Estrogens and the Psyche." *Clinical Obstetrics & Gynecology.* March 1981. Vol. 24, No. 1:219-29

Coulan, C.B. et al. "Chronic Anovulation Syndrome and Associated Neoplasia." *Obstetrics and Gynecology.* 1983. Vol. 61:403.

Council on Scientific Affairs. "Estrogen Replacement in the Menopause. *JAMA.* Vol. 249, No. 3:359-61.

Cramer, D.W. et al. "Factors Affecting the Association of Oral Contraceptives and Ovarian Cancer." *New England Journal of Medicine.* 1982. Vol. 307:1047-51.

Curtis, L.R., Curtis, G.B. and Beard, M.K. *My Body, My Decision.* The Body Press. 1986.

Davidson, B.J. et al. "Endogenous Cortisal and Sex Steroids in Patients with Osteoporotic Spinal Fractures." *Obstetrics and Gynecology.* 1983. Vol. 61:275-8.

Davis, M.R. "Osteoporosis Detection—Screening the Screens." *Contemporary OB/Gyn.* 1986. Vol. 28, No. 6:95-106.

Dawber, T.R. "The Framingham Study." Master's Thesis, Harvard University. 1980.

Dennerstein, L. "Psychologic Changes." *Menopause.* Yearbook Medical Publishers. 1987:115-

126.

Diczfalusy, E. "Menopause, Developing Countries and the 21st Century." *Menopause*. Year-book Medical Publishers. 1987:1-19.

DiSaia, Philip J. and William T. Creasman. *Clinical Gynecologic Oncology*. 2nd ed. C.V. Mosley. 1984.

Editorial. "Oral Contraceptives, The Good News." *JAMA*. 1983. Vol. 249,No. 12:1624-5.

Eichner, E.R. "Heart Disease Strikes Women Too." *Your Patient & Fitness*. October, 1990. 4:5-11.

Erlik, Y. et al. "Association of Waking Episodes with Menopausal Hot Flushes." *JAMA*. 1981. Vol. 245:1741-4.

Everson, R.B. "Effects of Passive Exposure to Smoking on Age at Menopause." *British Medical Journal*. 1986:298:792.

Flowers, C.E. et al. "Mechanisms of Uterine Bleeding in Postmenopausal Patients Receiving Estrogen Alone or with a Progestin." *Obstetrics and Gynecology*. 1983. Vol. 61, No. 2:135-43.

Friederich, M.A. "Advising the Woman at Menopause." *Contemporary OB/Gyn*. 1985. Vol. 24, No. 2:74-86.

Gallagher, J.C. et al. "Effect of Estrogen on Calcium Absorption and Serum Vitamin D Metabolites in Postmenopausal Osteoporosis." *Journal of Clinical Endocrinology & Metabolism*. 1980. Vol. 51:1359-63.

Gambrell, D. "The Use of Progestogens in Postmenopausal Women." *Menopausal Update*. 1985. Vol. 1:1-8.

Gambrell, D. et al. "Role of Estrogens and Progesterone in the Etiology and Prevention of Endometrial Cancer: Review." *American Journal of Obstetrics and Gynecology*. 1983. Vol. 146:696.

Gambrell, R.D. et al. "Decreased Incidence of Breast Cancer in Postmenopausal Estrogen-Progesterone Users." *Obstetrics and Gynecology*. 1983. Vol. 62:435.

Gold, E.B. "Smoking and the Menopause." *Menopause Management*. Nov. 1990. Vol. 3, No. 3:9-11.

Gordon, T. et al. "Menopause and Coronary Heart Disease: The Framingham Study." *Annals of Internal Medicine*. 1978. Vol. 89:157-61.

Hall, F.M. et al. "Bone Mineral Screening for Osteoporosis." *New England Journal of Medicine*. 1987. Vol. 316:212-4.

Hammond, C.B. "Estrogen Replacement Therapy: What the Future Holds." *American Journal of Obstetrics and Gynecology*. 1989. 161:1864-8.

Hammond, C.B. "Estrogen Therapy at Menopause." *Contemporary OB/Gyn*. 1983. Vol. 21:25-36.

Hammond, C.B. "Indications and Protocols for Estrogen Replacement Therapy." *Current Trends in Estrogen Replacement Therapy*. HP Publishing, 1986.

Hammond, M.G. "Managing Menopausal Signs and Symptoms." *Drug Therapy*. December 1984. 15-23.

Hazzard, W.R. "Estrogen Replacement and Cardiovascular Disease, Serum Lipids and Blood Pressure Effects." *American Journal of Obstetrics and Gynecology*. 1989. 161:1847-53.

Heaney, R.P., Recker, R.R. and Saville, P.D. "Calcium Balance and Calcium Requirements in Middle-Aged Women." *American Journal of Clinical Nutrition*. 1977. Vol. 30:1603-11.

Heaney, R.P., Recker, R.R. and Saville, P.D. "Menopausal Changes in Calcium Balance Performance." *Journal of Laboratory & Clinical Medicine*. 1978. Vol. 92:953.

Henderson, B.E. et al. "Estrogen Use and Cardiovascular Disease." *American Journal of Obstetrics and Gynecology*. 1986. Vol. 154:1181-6.

Hulka, B.S. "Effect of Exogenous Estrogen on Postmenopausal Women: The Epidemiologic Evidence." *Obstetrical and Gynecological Survey*. 1980. Vol. 35, No. 6:389-99.

Hulka, B.S. et al. "Protection Against Endometrial Carcinoma by Combination-Product Oral Contraceptive." *JAMA*. 1982. Vol. 247:475-7.

Jensen, C.F., Christiansen, C., et al. "Fracture Frequency and Bone Preservation in Postmenopausal Women Treated with Estrogen." *Obstetrics and Gynecology*. 1982. Vol. 60:493.

Jensen, J. et al. "Continuous Estrogen-Progesterone Treatment and Serum Lipoproteins in Postmenopausal Women." *British Journal of Obstetrics and Gynecology*. 1987. Vol.94:130-5.

Jensen, J. et al. "Long-Term Effects of Percutaneous Estrogens and Oral Progesterone on Serum Lipoproteins in Postmenopausal Women." *American Journal of Obstetrics and Gynecology*. 1987. Vol. 156:66-71.

Jensen, J., Christensen, C. and P. Rodtero. "Cigarette Smoking, Serum Estrogens and Bone Loss During Hormone-Replacement Therapy Early After Menopause." *New England Journal of Medicine*. 1985. Vol. 313:973-5.

Judd, H.L. et al. "Estrogen Replacement Therapy." *Obstetrics and Gynecology*. 1981. Vol. 58, No. 3:267-73.

Judd, H.L. "Effects of Estrogen Replacement on Hepatic Function." *Menopause*. Yearbook Medical Publishers. 1989. 237-251.

Kelsey, J.L. et al. "Risk Factors for Hip Fracture." *New England Journal of Medicine*. 1987. Vol. 316, No. 4:173-7.

Kerr, M.D. "Depression in Women after Late 30s Suggests Estrogen Deficit." *Internal Medicine News*. October 15, 1975.

Korenman, S.G. "Menopausal Endocrinology and Management." *Archives of Internal Medicine*. 1982. Vol. 142:1131-6.

Krauss, R.M. "Lipids and Lipoproteins in Postmenopausal Women." *Postgraduate Medicine*. Special Report, Sept. 1987:56-60.

Lane, C. et al. "How to Diagnose and Treat Osteoporosis after Menopause." *Contemporary OB/Gyn*. 1983:38-52.

Laufer, L.R. et al. "Estrogen Replacement Therapy by Transdermal Estradiol Administration." *American Journal of Obstetrics and Gynecology*. 1983. Vol. 146:533.

Laufer, L.R., et al. "Effect of Clonidine on Hot Flashes in Postmenopausal Women." *Obstetrics and Gynecology*. 1982. Vol. 60:583-6.

Lindsay, R. "Estrogen Replacement for Osteoporosis." *Current Trends in Estrogen Replacement Therapy*. HP Publishing Co. 1986.

Lindsay, R. "Identification of Bone Loss and Its Prevention by Sex Steroids." *Postgraduate Medicine*. Special Report, Sept. 1987:13-20.

Lindsay, R. "Pathophysiology of Bone Loss." *Drug Therapy Special Supplement*. Biomedical Information Corp. 1985.

Lindsay, R. et al. "Osteoporosis and Its Relationship to Estrogen." *Contemporary OB/Gyn*. 1984. Vol. 24, No. 1:201-24.

Lobo, R.A. et al. "Cardiovascular Effects of Estrogen Deprivation." *Postgraduate Medicine*. Special Report, Sept. 1987:29-38.

Lobo, R.A. "Cardiovascular Implications of Estrogen Replacement Therapy." *Obstetrics and Gynecology*. 1990. 185S-25S.

Lufkin, E.G. "Estrogen Efficacy and Side Effects in the Prevention and Treatment of Osteoporosis." *Current Perspective on Managing the Premenopausal and Postmenopausal Woman*. New York University Postgraduate Medical School. Dallas, TX. Dec. 8, 1990.

Lufkin, E.G., et al. "Estrogen Replacement Therapy: Current Recommendations." *Mayo Clinic Proceedings*. 1988:27:201-23.

Machal, L. "Postmenopausal Osteoporosis: New Approaches to Prevention." *Contemporary OB/Gyn*. 1982. Vol. 20:153-63.

Mandel, F.P. et al. "Effects of Progestins on Bone Metabolism in Postmenopausal Women." *Journal of Reproductive Medicine*. Vol. 27, No. 8:511-4.

Masters, W.H. and V.E. Johnson. *Human Sexual Response*. Little-Brown. 1966.

Masters, W.H. and V.E. Johnson. *Human Sexual Inadequacy*. Little-Brown. 1970.

Masters, W.H. and V.E. Johnson. "Sex and the Aging Process." *Journal of the American Geriatrics Society*. 1981. Vol. 29385-90.

Mathias, S. et al. "Drinking Coffee Raises Cholesterol in Women." *American Journal of Epidemiology*. 1985. Vol. 212:896-905.

Mead, P.B. and R.L. Sweet. "Looking for Chlamydia—and Finding It." *Contemporary OB/Gyn*. 1985. Vol. 25, No. 5:51-64.

Mischell, D.R. "Oral Contraception 1990: Taking Stock." *Dialogues in Contraception*. 1990. Vol. III, No. 1:1-3.

Mischell, D.R. "Contraceptive Practices in Older Women." *Obstetrics and Gynecology Audio Digest*. Oct. 5, 1990. 37, 19.

Morrison, J.C. et al. "The Use of Medroxyprogesterone Acetate for Relief of Climacteric Symptoms." *American Journal of Obstetrics and Gynecology*. 1980. Vol. 138:99.

Nachtigall, L.E. and Heilman, J.R. *Estrogen, The Facts Can Change Your Life*. Harper & Row.

1986.

Nachtigall, L.E. "Estrogen Replacement: Which Postmenopausal Women Benefit?" *Female Patient.* 1987. Vol. 12 (1987):72-86.

Nachtigall, L.E. et al. "Evaluating the Newly Menopausal Woman." *Contemporary OB/Gyn.* 1985. *Vol. 25, No. 5:68-92.*

Nachtigall, L.E. et al. "Estrogen Replacement Therapy: A 10-Year Prospective Study in the Relationship to Osteoporosis." *Obstetrics and Gynecology.* 1979. Vol. 53, No. 3:277-80.

Nachtigall, L.E. "Estrogen Replacement Therapy and Breast Cancer." *Current Perspective on Managing the Premenopausal and Postmenopausal Patient.* New York Postgraduate Medical School Conference. Dallas, TX. Dec. 8, 1990.

Nagamam, M. et al. "Treatment of Menopausal Hot Flashes with Transdermal Administration of Clonidine." *American Journal of Obstetrics and Gynecology.* 1987. Vol. 156:561-5.

Nagashima, T. "A High Prevalence of Chlamydial Cervicitis in Postmenopausal Women." *American Journal of Obstetrics and Gynecology.* 1987. Vol. 156:31-2.

Namburdiri, D.E. et al. "Sexuality After Menopause." *Female Patient.* 1987. Vol. 12:20-6.

Notelovitz, M. "Osteoporosis: A Decade's Findings in Prevention, Diagnosis and Treatment." *Female Patient.* 1986. Vol. 11:49-60.

Notelovitz, M. "Estrogen Replacement Therapy: Indications, Contraindications and Agent Selection." *American Journal of Obstetrics & Gynecology.* 1989. 161:1832-41.

Notelovitz, M. "Exercise and Osteoporosis." *Your Patient and Fitness.* 1987. Vol. 1, No. 4:10-6.

Olive, D.L. and Hammond, C.B. "The Menopause: Endocrinology, Physiology and Therapy." *Female Patient.* January 1986. Vol. 11:37-54.

"Osteoporosis." *National Institutes of Health Consensus Development Conference Statement.* 1984. Vol. 5, No. 3.

Padwick, M.L. et al. "Efficacy, Acceptability and Metabolic Effects of Transdermal Estradiol in the Management of Postmenopausal Women." *American Journal of Obstetrics and Gynecology.* 1985. Vol. 152:1092-99.

Peck, W.A. "The Nature of Osteoporosis." *Postgraduate Medicine.* Special Report, Sept. 1987:6-11.

"Pointers for Walkers." *University of California, Berkeley, Wellness Letter.* February 1987. Vol. 3, No. 5.

Pirie, L. and Curtis, L.R. *Pregnancy and Sports Fitness.* Fisher Books. 1987.

Powers, M.S. et al. "Pharmacokinetics and Pharmacodynamics of Transdermal Dosage Forms of 17B Estradiol: Comparison with Conventional Oral Estrogens Used for Hormone Replacement." *American Journal of Obstetrics and Gynecology.* 1985. Vol. 152:1099-1106.

Pritchard, J.A. et al. "The Human Ovary and Ovulation." *Williams Obstetrics.* 17th ed. Appleton-Century-Crafts. 1985.

Prough, S.G. "Continuous Estrogen/Progestin Therapy in Menopause." *American Journal of Obstetrics and Gynecology.* 1987. Vol. 157:149-53.

Quigley, M.E. et al. "Estrogen Therapy Arrests Bone Loss in Elderly Women." *American Journal of Obstetrics and Gynecology.* 1987. Vol. 156:1516-23.

Ravnikar, V.A. "Compliance with Hormone Therapy." *American Journal of Obstetrics and Gynecology.* 1987. Vol. 156:1332-4.

Ravnikar, V.A., et al. "Hormone Therapy for Menopausal Sleep Problems." *Contemporary Ob/Gyn.* Oct. 1982. Vol. 20:71-93.

Ravnikar, V.A. et al. "Hormone Therapy for Menopausal Sleep Problems?" *Contemporary OB/Gyn.* Oct. 1982. Vol. 20:71-93.

Richart, R.M. et al. "Detecting Endometrial Cancer and Precursor Lesions." *Contemporary OB/Gyn.* Vol. 21 (1983):231-47.

Ross, R.J. and Henderson, B.E. "Estrogen Replacement in the Prevention of Cardiovascular Disease. *Current Trends in Estrogen Replacement Therapy.* HP Publishing. 1986.

Ross, R.K. et al. "Menopausal Estrogen Therapy and Protection from Death from Ischemic Heart Disease." *Lancet.* 1981. Vol. 1:858-60.

Roy, A. "Hepatic Effects of Hormone Therapy." *Postgraduate Medicine* Special Report. Sept. 1987:39-47.

Saville, P.D. "Postmenopausal Osteoporosis and Estrogens: Who Should Be Treated and Why." 1984. Vol. 75, No. 2:135-143.

Schiff, I., et al. "Oral Medoxyprogesterone in the Treatment of Postmenopausal Symptoms." *JAMA.* 1980. Vol. 244:1443-5.

Schiff, I. and Ryan, K.J. "Benefits of Estrogen Replacement." *Obstetrical & Gynecological Survey.* 1980. Vol. 35., No. 6:400-9.

Semmens, J.P. and Wagner, C. "Estrogen Deprivation and Vaginal Function in Postmenopausal Women." *JAMA.* 1982. Vol. 248:445-8.

Semmens, J.P. et al. "Effects of Estrogen Therapy on Vaginal Physiology during Menopause." *Obstetrics and Gynecology.* 1985. Vol. 69:15.

Semmens, J.P. "Postmenopausal Vaginal Physiology—Effects of Estrogen Deprivation on Sexual Relations." *Clinical Practice in Sexuality.* 1986. Vol. 3., No. 7:10-7.

Shangold, M.D. "Advising Women about Exercise: What to Tell Your Patients." *Female Patient.* 1987. Vol. 12:57-65.

Shangold, M.M. "Exercise in the Menopausal Woman." *Obstetrics and Gynecology.* 1990. Vol. 75:53S.

Sharf, M. et al. "Lipid and Lipoprotein Levels Following Pure Estradiol Implantation in Postmenopausal Women." *Gynecologogic and Obstetric Investigations.* Vol. 19:207-212.

Simsen, D.A. et al. "Endometrial Findings and Asymptomatic Postmenopausal Women on Exogenous Estrogens—A Preliminary Report." *Gynecology Oncology.* 1981. Vol. 11:56-63.

Sorrel, D.M. "Sexuality and Menopause." *Obstetrics and Gynecology.* 1990. 75:26S.

Spellacy, W.N. "Menopause, Estrogen Treatment and Carbohydrate Metabolism." *Menopause.* Yearbook Medical Publishers. 1987. 256-258.

Speroff, L. "Estrogen Replacement Today: A Preventive Health Care Issue." *Current Trends in Estrogen Replacement Therapy.* HP Publishing. 1986.

Speroff, L. et al. "Sexuality in Older Women." *Contemporary OB/Gyn.* 1986. Vol. 27:212.

Steingold, K.A. et al. "Treatment of Hot Flashes with Transdermal Estradiol Administration." *Journal of Clinical Endocrinology & Metabolism.* 1985. Vol. 61:627.

Stevenson, J.C. "Etiology of Osteoporosis." *Drug Therapy Special Supplement.* Biomedical Information Corp. 1985.

Stevenson, J.C. "Pathogenesis, Prevention and Treatment of Osteoporosis." *Obstetrics and Gynecology.* 1990. 75:36S.

Storm, T., et al. "Effect of Intermittent Cyclical Etidronate Therapy on Bone Mass and Fracture Rate in Women with Postmenopausal Osteoporosis." *New England Journal of Medicine.* 1990. Vol. 322:1265-1271.

Symposium. "ERT—Who to Treat and How." *Contemporary OB/Gyn.* 1987. Vol. 29, No. 4:179-93.

Tataryn, I.V. et al. "LH, FSH and Skin Temperature During the Menopausal Hot Flash." *Journal of Clinical Endocrinology & Metabolism.* 1979. Vol. 49:152-4.

Taylor, R.B. "Osteoporosis Prevention and Management." *Female Patient.* Vol. 10:20-31.

Teran, A. "Estrogen Replacement Therapy for the Menopause: What to Do About It?" *Obstetrics and Gynecology Forum.* 1987. Vol. 1, No. 5:5-11.

Townsend, M. "Management of Breast Cancer." *Clinical Symposia* (CIBA-Geigy). 1987. Vol. 39, No. 4:3-32.

Upton, C.V. "Goals and Methods of Hormone Replacement after Menopause." *Contemporary OB/Gyn.* 1985. Vol. 25, No. 1:75-83.

Utian, W.H. "Biosynthesis and Physiologic Effects of Estrogen and Pathophysiologic Effects of Estrogen Deficiency: A Review." *American Journal of Obstetrics and Gynecology.* 1989. Vol. 161:1828-31.

Utian, W.H. "Current Perspectives in Management of the Menopausal and Postmenopausal Patient: Introduction." *Obstetrics and Gynecology.* 1990. 75:1S.

Vandenbrouche, J.P. et al. "Noncontraceptive Hormones and Rheumatoid Arthritis in Perimenopausal and Postmenopausal Women." *JAMA.* 1986. Vol. 255:1299-1303.

Vandenbroucke, J.P. "Oral Contraceptives and Rheumatoid Arthritis in Perimenopausal and Postmenopausal Women." *JAMA.* 1986. Vol. 255:1299-1303.

Wasserstein, A. "The Calcium Stone Former with Osteoporosis." *JAMA.* 1987. Vol. 257:2215.

Watts, N.B., et al. "Intermittent Cyclical Etidronate Treatment of Postmenopausal Osteoporosis." *New England Journal of Medicine.* 1990. 323:73-9.

Whitehead, M.I. et al. "Endometrial Responses to Transdermal Estradiol in Postmenopausal

Women." *American Journal of Obstetrics and Gynecology.* 1985. Vol. 152:1079-84.

Williams, A.R. et al. "Effect of Weight, Smoking and Estrogen Use in the Risk of Hip and Forearm Fractures in Postmenopausal Women." *Obstetrics and Gynecology.* 1982. Vol. 60:695-8.

Woolf, A.D. et al. "Osteoporosis, An Update on Management." *Drugs.* 1984. Vol. 28:565-76.

Ziel, H.K. and Finkle, W.D. "Increased Risk of Endometrial Carcinoma Among Users of Congugated Estrogens." *New England Journal of Medicine.* 1975. Vol. 293:1167-70.

Index